A Vegan Taste of Central America

Also by Linda Majzlik

A Vegan Taste of Central America

Linda Majzlik

Jon Carpenter

Our books may be ordered from bookshops or (post free) from
Jon Carpenter Publishing, Alder House, Market Street, Charlbury,
England OX7 3PH

Credit card orders may be phoned or faxed to 01689 870437
or 01608 811969

First published in 2005 by
Jon Carpenter Publishing
Alder House, Market Street, Charlbury, Oxfordshire OX7 3PH
☎ 01608 811969

© Linda Majzlik 2005

Illustrations © Amanda Henriques   Cover design by Sarah Tyzack

ISBN 1 897766 98 X

Printed in England by J W Arrowsmith, Bristol

CONTENTS

Main courses

Accompaniments

Snacks

Rice

Salads

Salsas and sauces

Breads

Drinks

INTRODUCTION

Known collectively as Central America, the seven compact countries of Belize, Costa Rica, El Salvador, Guatemala, Honduras, Nicaragua and Panama occupy the thin strip of land that connects the vast continents of North and South America. Extending for 1,200 miles from Mexico in the northwest to Colombia in the southeast, this isthmus is barely 300 miles across at its widest point in the north and narrows to just 75 miles in the south. The whole area is roughly a quarter of the size of Mexico and it is home to around 27 million people.

The rich culture of the Mayas, an American Indian people of Yucatan, Belize and North Guatemala, flourished between AD 250 and 900 and the ruins of their huge stone temples, shaped like pyramids, are now a big tourist attraction. Their descendants still live on the Yucatan peninsula, where they uphold the traditions and culture of their ancestors and speak the Mayan language. The official language in most of Central America is Spanish, although in the former British colony Belize it is English.

Lying between the Caribbean Sea and the Pacific Ocean, the region has a wide variety of climatic conditions, which can range in relatively small areas from tropical to temperate and cool, depending on the height of the land. Northeasterly winds bring heavy rainfall throughout the year on the Caribbean side, while only seasonal rains fall on the Pacific coastal plains. Severe weather conditions such as droughts, tropical storms, floods and hurricanes cause extensive damage at times and being situated where four tectonic plates converge, the area is also seriously affected by earthquakes and volcanic eruptions. The region boasts a diversity of spectacular landscapes, such as dense tropical rainforests, high mountainous peaks, rugged volcanic ridges, low-lying coastal plains, vast lakes and lagoons and long sandy beaches.

The low-lying plains with their rich volcanic soils offer some of the best growing conditions for all kinds of fruits, vegetables and grains, while the volcanic uplands are ideally suited to growing coffee, a major export. Corn and beans, the mainstays of the diet, can be cultivated at all altitudes and evidence has been found that these two staples have been grown in the region for around 7,000 and 4,000 years respectively. In fact, many of the foods that sustained the native American Indians centuries ago are as important today as they were then. Along with corn and beans the ancient diet was also based on avocados, cassavas, chillies, peppers, squashes, tomatoes, various types of potato and a wide variety of soft fruits.

The Spanish 'discovered' the region in the 16th century and subsequently took control for more than 300 years. During this time they introduced new crops such as wheat, sugar, rice, citrus fruits and bananas and also took many of the native American foods back with them to Europe and to other parts of the world. In more recent times thousands of Afro-Caribbeans arrived to help build the railways and the Panama Canal and to work on the vast sugar and banana plantations. These workers brought ingredients such as yams, okras and coconuts with them and all these new introductions have now been absorbed into the native cuisine.

As is the tradition in all Latin American countries, the main meal of the day is generally eaten at midday. It can consist of soup or a selection of little savoury appetisers, followed by the main course, usually accompanied by a grain dish, salad, salsa, vegetable dish and tortillas or bread. All foods are served in communal dishes for diners to help themselves to and it is considered rude to take food and leave it uneaten on the plate, as wasting food is frowned upon. Typically for dessert fresh fruit is served, although more elaborate dishes are made for special occasions. Fruit drinks are often served with the meal and coffee or hot chocolate are favourites to round off a meal.

A much lighter meal is served in the evening and might simply consist of leftovers from the midday meal, as no food is ever wasted. Breakfast is very often savoury-based rather than sweet and commonly served dishes include rice and beans, soup, tortillas stuffed with leftovers or thick porridge made from cornmeal and flavoured with chillies. Both sweet and savoury snacks are popular throughout the day and are typically served with coffee or hot chocolate.

Central American cuisine, with its mixture of native, Spanish and Afro-Caribbean influences, offers a very homely style of cooking with lots of easy-to-prepare dishes based on fresh wholesome ingredients. You may not want to go as far as eating chilli-flavoured porridge for breakfast, but you may well want to experiment and incorporate some new and flavourful recipes into your repertoire of vegan dishes.

THE VEGAN CENTRAL AMERICAN STORECUPBOARD

Many of the staple vegetables used in the region such as cassava, chayote, plantain, potato, squash and sweet potato keep very well when stored in a dark, dry, airy cupboard. These can be combined with other seasonal produce or items from the storecupboard to produce some authentic Central American dishes.

Amaranth Native to Central and South America, amaranth is a highly nutritious seed which is treated as a grain and used in various savoury recipes. The leaves of the plant are eaten as a vegetable and it is estimated that each plant, which can grow up to 7 feet tall, can produce up to 60,000 seeds. When cooked, amaranth has a sticky texture and a pleasant nutty flavour.

Beans A fundamental staple in all Central American countries, beans are an excellent source of nutrition and they are used in countless recipes or simply eaten as an accompaniment. Black, pinto and red kidney are all popular varieties and in most households are cooked in bulk and eaten with every meal. Cooking a large quantity of beans at the same time is a good idea, as they can be frozen sucessfully. However, tinned beans make a useful standby.

Capers The small green flower buds from a trailing bush, capers have a piquant taste and are sold preserved in either vinegar or brine. They are occasionally used as an ingredient and for garnishing.

'Cheese' Various recipes require 'cheese' either as an ingredient or as a topping and vegan 'Cheddar'-type versions are used here.

Chickpeas Creamy, nutty-flavoured chickpeas are a rich source of protein, fibre, vitamins and minerals. They are popular for serving cold in salads.

Chillies Fresh chillies are a crucial ingredient in Central American cuisine and numerous varieties are grown and used in the region. Some of the most popular types are jalapeño, habanero and tabasco. Bottled jalapeño chillies are often used as an ingredient and for garnishing or are simply served in bowls as a condiment. Fresh chillies keep well in the fridge for 7-10 days.

Chocolate Cocoa beans, the seeds of the cacao tree which is native to Mexico, were so highly prized by ancient civilisations that they were used as currency. Hot chocolate drinks are very popular in Central America, as are chocolate-flavoured desserts and cakes. An ever-increasing range of vegan chocolate bars is readily available.

Cocoa powder Made from roasted and ground cocoa beans, cocoa powder is used in various sweet recipes.

Coconut Not a true nut, but the fruit of the coconut palm which thrives in hot tropical regions. Used in various forms, coconut adds richness and flavour to sweet and savoury dishes.

Creamed This is pure fresh coconut flesh shaped into a vacuum-packed block. Once opened the block needs to be kept in the fridge and used within a couple of weeks. For longer storage, grate the block and freeze.

Desiccated The dried flesh of the coconut, available sweetened, unsweetened, toasted or plain.

Flaked Flakes of dried coconut flesh can be used to garnish both sweet and savoury dishes. Lightly toasting the flakes enhances the flavour.

Milk A thick rich liquid made from pressed coconut flesh, this is available tinned or in cartons. Reduced-fat and thin versions are also available. Coconut milk can also be made by dissolving 4oz/100g grated creamed coconut in 20 fl.oz/600ml hot water. Any unused coconut milk can be frozen.

Cornflour A very fine starchy white flour milled from maize. It is sometimes known as cornstarch and is used for thickening sweet and savoury sauces.

Cornmeal Ground maize, which is milled in various grades from fine to coarse. Also known as maizemeal, it is regularly used to make cornbread and as an ingredient in numerous sweet and savoury recipes.

'Cream' Soya cream is used here in ice cream desserts.

'Cream cheese' Excellent vegan versions made from soya are available from health food shops and supermarkets. It is used here combined with other ingredients to make savoury spreads and toppings.

Dijon mustard A mixture of ground mustard seeds and spices, Dijon mustard has quite a mild flavour and is a favourite ingredient in salad dressings.

Ginger root Not widely used in savoury dishes, but enjoyed as a flavouring in fruit drinks and certain desserts. Fresh root ginger will keep in the fridge for up to 10 days or can be cut into portions, wrapped individually in foil or cling film and frozen.

Golden syrup Sweet and delicate in taste, this thick syrup is made from molasses residue that has been clarified. It is used in cake recipes and helps bind mixtures together.

Hearts of palm Also known as palm hearts or palmito in Central America, these are the edible shoots of a variety of palm tree. They are not usually available fresh outside the region, but they can be readily found tinned and simply need to be drained and rinsed before use. Hearts of palm have a fresh delicate flavour and are a popular ingredient in salads, rice dishes and cold soups. They are also chopped or sliced and used as a garnish.

Herbs Compared to other cuisines, only a few herbs are used regularly in Central American recipes.

Coriander Undoubtedly the most popular herb throughout the region, coriander is always used fresh and never dried. It has a unique flavour and is used both as an ingredient and as a garnish.

Oregano Sometimes referred to as wild marjoram, oregano is a small-leafed herb that has a natural affinity with tomatoes.

Parsley This universally popular herb is used both as an ingredient and for garnishing and the flat-leafed variety is preferred.

Thyme A small-leafed, highly aromatic herb which is widely used in all Central American countries.

Lemon and lime juice Citrus fruits are grown in several Central American countries and fresh lemon and lime juice is used in various savoury and sweet recipes.

Masa harina Specially prepared fine flour, which is milled from dried maize and used to make corn tortillas.

Mayonnaise Some excellent egg-free versions are available in health food shops and increasingly in supermarkets. Mayonnaise is used in some salads, but more often in dips.

Parmesan An authentic-tasting vegan version made from soya is available from health food stores and some supermarkets. It is sometimes used as a garnish or topping and is the essential filling for picos, savoury little bread triangles.

Peanuts Native to Mexico, peanuts, or groundnuts as they are also called, are an excellent source of protein, minerals and vitamins. They are enjoyed as a snack or roasted and ground and used in stews. Chopped roasted peanuts are used as a garnish.

Peanut butter Smooth or crunchy versions can be used in sweet and savoury recipes.

Pumpkin seeds These pale green seeds are a very rich source of iron and zinc. They are enjoyed as a snack and are an essential ingredient in pepian dishes, where they are roasted and ground and used as the basis for a savoury sauce.

Quinoa Pronounced 'keen-wa', this protein-rich, gluten-free 'grain' is native to Central and South America, where it was regarded as holy in ancient times and referred to as the 'mother grain'. Although not a true grain it is treated as such and as it contains all eight essential amino acids it is a complete source of protein. It is eaten plainly cooked as an accompaniment to stews or mixed with other ingredients in various recipes. The plant is in fact related to spinach and in Central American countries the leaves are also eaten, either raw or cooked. The raw 'grain' must be rinsed thoroughly in water before cooking to remove the bitter-tasting saponins which act as a natural insect repellent.

Rice Introduced by the Spanish in the 16th century, rice is now a staple food all over Central America. It is commonly combined with beans and in some countries it is served with every meal. Long grain rice is the most popular variety. Sweetened rice pudding is a favourite dessert and variations are found in all the countries.

Sesame seeds These tiny protein- and calcium-rich seeds are roasted and ground and used in pepian dishes. The whole seeds are also sprinkled on breads and some savoury dishes before baking.

Soya milk Unsweetened soya milk has been used in both sweet and savoury recipes.

Spices These are bought whole and ground at home as and when required.

Allspice Tasting of a mixture of cinnamon, cloves and nutmeg, allspice is the dried berry of an evergreen tree grown in the region. It is used extensively in sweet and savoury dishes.

Black pepper An essential seasoning in savoury dishes. Coarsely-ground black peppercorns are preferred to ready-ground pepper.

Cayenne pepper The dried fruit of a hot red pepper, deep red in colour and very pungent. Cayenne is used to add 'heat' to a dish.

Cinnamon Used both as sticks and ground, cinnamon has a warm sweet flavour and is used regularly in sweet dishes.

Cloves The dried buds of an evergreen tree, which are valued for their anaesthetic and antiseptic properties. Whole cloves are a favourite flavouring for sweet rice puddings.

Coriander The dried seed of a plant belonging to the parsley family, coriander has a mild, sweet, orangey flavour and is used ground in various savoury dishes.

Cumin Used both as seeds and ground, cumin has a strong, earthy flavour and is used in all kinds of savoury dishes.

Paprika A dried and ground sweet red pepper which adds colour and a mild sweet flavour to savoury dishes, especially those containing tomatoes.

Sweetcorn A basic staple which has been grown in the region for at least 7,000 years. Maize, which is a good source of carbohydrates, fibre, vitamins and minerals, finds its way in some shape or form into all kinds of dishes, from starters to desserts, cakes and drinks. Fresh sweetcorn is preferred, but frozen or tinned corn may be substituted.

Tabasco sauce A very hot piquant sauce, made from tabasco chillies which have been steeped in vinegar and matured in casks for several years.

Textured vegetable protein A nutritious and versatile soya product which readily absorbs the flavours of other ingredients. The natural minced variety is used here in various savoury recipes.

Tinned tomatoes Crushed tinned tomatoes are sometimes used in preference to fresh if a stronger tomato flavour is required.

Tomato purée Used to strengthen the flavour of and add colour to tomato-based dishes.

Vegetable oils Corn, sunflower, groundnut and olive oils are all regularly used, with olive oil generally being reserved for making salad dressings and salsas and the occasional cooked dish in which the flavour is desired.

Vegetable stock The liquid that is left over from cooking beans is always used as vegetable stock. If this is not available, Central American cooks often use stock cubes. Check ingredients labels on vegetable stock cubes, as many contain animal-derived ingredients.

Vinegar White wine vinegar is favoured for making salad dressings and for using in salsas.

Yoghurt Used in dips and sometimes swirled into soups, plain soya yoghurt makes an excellent substitute.

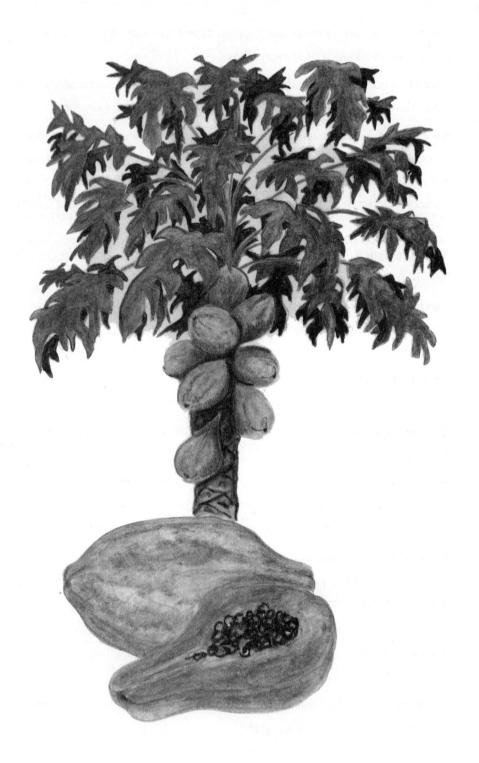

SOUPS

An interesting and imaginative assortment of hot and cold soups are enjoyed in all Central American countries, served both as starters before a main course and as snacks throughout the day. Although the soups detailed below are all made from scratch, they give a good idea of the varieties created by Central American cooks, who frequently make soups with leftovers from previous meals and use the cooking liquid from beans as stock when available. Stale tortillas are often chopped up and added to soups and chunks of bread are served alongside for mopping up.

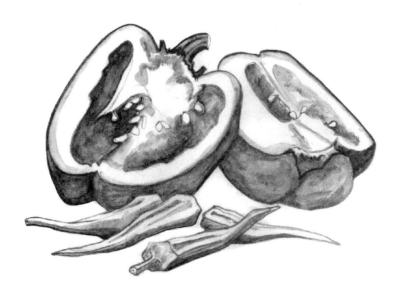

Black bean soup (serves 4)

8oz/225g cooked black beans

6oz/175g potato, peeled and finely chopped

1 red onion, peeled and finely chopped

1 small red chilli, deseeded and finely chopped

2 garlic cloves, crushed

1 dessertspoon olive oil

2 tablespoons finely chopped fresh coriander

20 fl.oz/600ml vegetable stock

black pepper

Fry the onion, chilli and garlic in the oil for 5 minutes, then add the remaining ingredients and stir well. Bring to the boil, cover and simmer, stirring occasionally, for about 10 minutes until the potato is done. Allow to cool slightly before blending the soup smooth. Return to the rinsed out pan and reheat.

Avocado and tomato soup (serves 4)

1 medium avocado, peeled, stoned and chopped

8oz/225g tomatoes, skinned and chopped

1 small onion, peeled and chopped

1 green chilli, deseeded and chopped

1 dessertspoon olive oil

1 rounded tablespoon finely chopped fresh parsley

20 fl.oz/600ml vegetable stock

black pepper

plain soya yoghurt

Soften the onion and chilli in the oil, add the tomatoes, parsley and stock and season with black pepper. Bring to the boil, cover and simmer for 3 minutes. Allow to cool slightly, then blend with the avocado until smooth. Pour the soup back into the cleaned pan and reheat. Ladle the soup into serving bowls and garnish with a swirl of plain yoghurt.

Sweet potato, peanut and corn soup (serves 4)

1lb/450g sweet potatoes, peeled and diced

4oz/100g sweetcorn kernels

1 onion, peeled and finely chopped

1 small red chilli, deseeded and finely chopped

2 rounded tablespoons peanut butter

1 dessertspoon corn oil

½ teaspoon ground coriander

½ teaspoon ground cumin

black pepper

24 fl.oz/725ml vegetable stock

chopped roasted peanuts

Fry the onion and chilli in the oil in a large pan until softened. Add the sweet potatoes, coriander, cumin and stock and season with black pepper. Stir well and bring to the boil, cover and simmer for 10 minutes. Put in the sweetcorn and simmer for 2 minutes more, then add the peanut butter and stir around for a couple of minutes until well combined. Remove from the heat and mash the soup lightly before ladling it into bowls. Garnish with chopped peanuts.

Okra and amaranth soup (serves 4)

8oz/225g okras, topped and cut into ½ inch/1cm diagonal slices

8oz/225g tomatoes, skinned and chopped

3oz/75g amaranth

1 red onion, peeled and finely chopped

1 red chilli, deseeded and finely chopped

2 garlic cloves, crushed

1 dessertspoon corn oil

2 tablespoons finely chopped fresh coriander

26 fl.oz/775ml vegetable stock

1 teaspoon paprika

¼ teaspoon ground allspice

black pepper

grated vegan 'cheese' (optional)

Heat the oil in a large pan and soften the onion, chilli and garlic. Add the tomatoes and cook until pulpy, then stir in the stock, amaranth, paprika and allspice and season with black pepper. Bring to the boil, cover and simmer for 15 minutes. Now add the okra and coriander and simmer for a further 10 minutes until tender. Sprinkle each bowl of soup with grated 'cheese' if wished.

Roasted red pepper soup (serves 4)

1lb/450g red peppers

6oz/175g tomatoes, halved

1 red onion, peeled and chopped

1 red chilli, deseeded and chopped

2 garlic cloves, crushed

1 dessertspoon olive oil

18 fl.oz/525ml vegetable stock

1 rounded dessertspoon tomato purée

1 teaspoon paprika

½ teaspoon dried thyme

black pepper

finely sliced spring onions

Roast the red peppers and tomatoes under a hot grill until the skins blister on the peppers and the tomatoes are pulpy. Carefully remove the skins, stalks, membranes and seeds from the peppers and chop the flesh. Remove the skins from the tomatoes and put them in a blender with the chopped pepper.

Fry the onion, chilli and garlic in the oil until soft, then add to the blender together with the stock, tomato purée, paprika and thyme. Season with black pepper and blend until smooth. Pour into a saucepan and bring to the boil, stirring frequently, then ladle into bowls and garnish with sliced spring onions.

Corn and quinoa soup (serves 4)

12oz/350g sweetcorn kernels

3oz/75g quinoa

1 onion, peeled and finely chopped

2 garlic cloves, crushed

1 red chilli, deseeded and finely chopped

1 dessertspoon corn oil

2 rounded tablespoons finely chopped fresh coriander

black pepper

20 fl.oz/600ml vegetable stock

10 fl.oz/300ml water

grated vegan 'cheese' (optional)

Heat the oil in a large pan and fry the onion, garlic and chilli until softened. Add the quinoa and stock and bring to the boil, then cover and simmer for 10 minutes. Meanwhile blend 8oz/225g of the sweetcorn smooth with the water. Add this mixture to the pan together with the rest of the sweetcorn kernels and the coriander. Season with black pepper and bring back to the boil. Simmer for another 10 minutes, stirring occasionally. Ladle the soup into serving bowls and sprinkle with grated 'cheese' if liked.

Tomato and rice soup (serves 4)

8oz/225g ripe tomatoes, skinned and chopped

4oz/100g long grain rice

1 red onion, peeled and finely chopped

1 small red chilli, deseeded and finely chopped

2 garlic cloves, crushed

1 tablespoon olive oil

1 rounded dessertspoon tomato purée

1 teaspoon cumin seeds

1 rounded tablespoon finely chopped fresh coriander

black pepper
20 fl.oz/600ml vegetable stock
chopped green olives

Cook the rice, then drain and set aside. Fry the onion, chilli and garlic in the oil until soft. Add the tomatoes and cumin seeds and cook for a few minutes until the tomatoes are soft, then mash them with the back of a spoon. Put in the cooked rice, tomato purée, coriander and stock, season with black pepper and stir well. Bring to the boil, cover and simmer for 10 minutes, stirring occasionally. Serve garnished with chopped olives.

Green vegetable and tortilla soup (serves 4)

24 tortilla chips (see page 31)
4oz/100g green pepper, chopped
4oz/100g green beans, topped, tailed and cut into 1 inch/2.5cm
    lengths
4oz/100g broccoli, chopped
1 avocado, peeled, stoned and halved
1 onion, peeled and chopped
1 green chilli, deseeded and finely chopped
1 garlic clove, crushed
1 dessertspoon corn oil
18 fl.oz/525ml vegetable stock
1 teaspoon dried oregano
black pepper
chopped fresh parsley

Fry the onion, chilli and garlic in the oil until softened, then add the green pepper, beans, broccoli, vegetable stock and oregano. Season with black pepper and bring to the boil. Cover and simmer, stirring occasionally, for 15 minutes. Meanwhile mash one half of the avocado and dice the other half. Add the mashed avocado to the soup together with the tortilla chips, stir well and bring back to the boil. Simmer for 2-3 minutes, then ladle the soup into bowls and garnish with the diced avocado and some chopped parsley.

Tomato, okra and baby corn soup (serves 4)

8oz/225g tomatoes, skinned and chopped

6oz/175g okras, topped, and cut into ½ inch/1cm diagonal slices

6oz/175g baby corn, cut into ½ inch/1cm diagonal slices

1 red onion, peeled and finely chopped

1 green chilli, deseeded and finely chopped

2 garlic cloves, crushed

1 tablespoon olive oil

1 tablespoon tomato purée

1 rounded teaspoon dried thyme

black pepper

16 fl.oz/475ml vegetable stock

grated vegan 'cheese' (optional)

Heat the oil in a large pan and soften the onion and chilli. Add the tomatoes and cook until pulpy. Stir in the stock, okras, corn, garlic, tomato purée and thyme. Season with black pepper and bring to the boil, then cover and simmer for about 15 minutes, stirring occasionally, until cooked. Serve sprinkled with grated 'cheese' if wished.

Mixed bean soup (serves 4)

8oz/225g green beans, topped, tailed and cut into 1 inch/2.5cm lengths

8oz/225g cooked mixed beans (e.g. pinto, red kidney, black)

8oz/225g tomatoes, skinned and chopped

1 red onion, peeled and finely chopped

2 garlic cloves, crushed

1 tablespoon tomato purée

1 tablespoon olive oil

1 teaspoon dried thyme

½ teaspoon cayenne pepper

black pepper

20 fl.oz/600ml vegetable stock

finely chopped fresh parsley

grated vegan 'cheese' (optional)

Fry the onion and garlic in the oil in a large pan until soft. Add the tomatoes and gently cook until pulpy, then stir in the stock, green and mixed beans, tomato purée, thyme and cayenne pepper and season with black pepper. Bring to the boil, cover and simmer, stirring occasionally, for about 15 minutes until the green beans are tender. Ladle the soup into serving bowls and sprinkle with chopped parsley and, if liked, grated 'cheese'.

Chilled avocado soup (serves 4)

1 large avocado, peeled, stoned and chopped

1 onion, peeled and chopped

1 green chilli, deseeded and chopped

1 dessertspoon olive oil

1 dessertspoon lime juice

dash of Tabasco sauce

22 fl.oz/650ml vegetable stock

black pepper

finely chopped fresh coriander

2 spring onions, trimmed and finely sliced

Soften the onion and chilli in the oil. Transfer to a blender and add the avocado, lime juice, Tabasco sauce and stock. Season with black pepper and blend smooth. Refrigerate until cold, then stir the soup and serve garnished with chopped coriander and sliced spring onions.

Chilled cucumber and hearts of palm soup (serves 4)

14oz/400g tin hearts of palm, drained, rinsed and chopped

8oz/225g cucumber, chopped

6 spring onions, trimmed and chopped

16 fl.oz/475ml cold vegetable stock

2 tablespoons lemon juice

2 teaspoons dried parsley

black pepper

plain soya yoghurt

Put the hearts of palm, cucumber, spring onions, stock, lemon juice and parsley in a blender, season with black pepper and blend until smooth. Chill for a few hours, then stir and ladle into serving bowls. Garnish each bowl of soup with a swirl of yoghurt before serving.

APPETISERS

A selection of savoury appetisers is usually offered before the main course and these can range from easily prepared dips and spreads for tortillas and breads to more elaborate little savoury tarts such as canastitas. These are so popular in some Central American countries that large packs of ready-made bases or 'little baskets', which is what canastitas means, are readily available, so that only a filling needs to be added at home. As well as the one given below, other typical fillings are vegetable picadillo, refried beans and avocado and 'cream cheese' spread. Alternatively, the bases can be baked blind until golden brown and filled with a salsa.

The toppings for tostadas can also be varied according to what is available and these too are equally good topped with refried beans, any of the salsas or finely chopped salad ingredients. Bowls of roasted peanuts and pumpkin seeds are also commonly served as appetisers, as are thinly sliced sweet potato, plaintain and cassava, fried until crispy and golden.

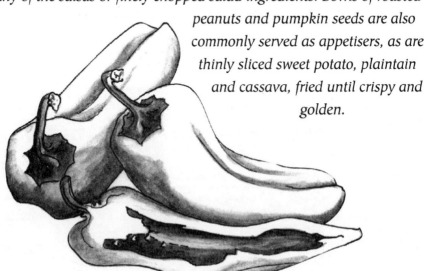

Avocado dip (serves 4)

1 large avocado, peeled, stoned and mashed

2 rounded tablespoons vegan mayonnaise

1 tablespoon lemon juice

1 garlic clove, crushed

1 small red chilli, deseeded and finely chopped

2 spring onions, trimmed and finely chopped

black pepper

Mix the ingredients until well combined. Serve with tortilla chips or crudités.

Avocado and pumpkin seed dip (serves 4)

1 medium avocado, peeled, stoned and mashed

2oz/50g pumpkin seeds, roasted and ground

1 tablespoon lime juice

4 rounded tablespoons plain soya yoghurt

black pepper

Combine all the ingredients well. Spoon into a serving dish and serve with tortilla chips or crudités.

Tortilla chips (serves 4)

5 4 inch/10cm corn tortillas (see page 89)

corn oil

chilli powder

Cut each tortilla into 6 triangles and deep fry in hot oil for a few minutes until golden. Drain on kitchen paper and sprinkle with chilli powder.

Tostadas (makes 8)

8 4 inch/10cm corn tortillas (see page 89)

corn oil

2oz/50g vegan 'cream cheese'

2oz/50g tinned hearts of palm, drained, rinsed and finely chopped

2 spring onions, trimmed and finely chopped

1 teaspoon dried parsley

black pepper

tomato and chilli salsa (see page 84)

1 small avocado, peeled, stoned and diced

finely chopped fresh coriander

Put the 'cream cheese', hearts of palm, spring onions and parsley in a large bowl, season with black pepper and mix thoroughly.

Briefly fry the corn tortillas in hot oil, then drain on kitchen paper. Spread each tortilla with some of the 'cream cheese' mixture and top with a little tomato and chilli salsa. Garnish with diced avocado and chopped coriander.

Fried potato and corn cakes (makes 8)

8oz/225g potatoes, peeled

4oz/100g sweetcorn kernels

1 small onion, peeled and grated

2oz/50g cornmeal

1 rounded tablespoon finely chopped fresh parsley

black pepper

3 tablespoons soya milk

corn oil

Cook the potatoes, drain and mash. Blanch the sweetcorn kernels, then drain and add to the potato together with the onion, parsley, cornmeal and soya milk. Season with black pepper and mix well. Take rounded tablespoonfuls of the mixture, roll into balls and flatten these to about ½ inch/1cm thick. Shallow fry the cakes in hot oil for a few minutes on each side until golden brown. Drain on kitchen paper and serve hot with a salsa and salad garnish.

Chickpea and red pepper ceviche (serves 4)

10oz/300g cooked chickpeas

6oz/175g red peppers, finely chopped

2 garlic cloves, crushed

½ small red onion, peeled and finely chopped

1 tablespoon olive oil

2 dessertspoons lemon juice

1 rounded dessertspoon tomato purée

1 dessertspoon white wine vinegar

1 rounded teaspoon dried oregano

¼ teaspoon cayenne pepper

black pepper

finely chopped fresh parsley

finely grated lemon peel

Combine the chickpeas, red pepper, garlic and onion in a large bowl. Mix the olive oil with the lemon juice, tomato purée, vinegar, oregano and cayenne pepper and add. Season with black pepper and toss thoroughly. Cover and chill for a few hours. Serve in individual bowls, garnished with parsley and lemon peel.

Savoury mince and black bean balls (serves 4)

4oz/100g cooked black beans, mashed

2oz/50g natural minced textured vegetable protein

2oz/50g breadcrumbs

1 onion, peeled and finely chopped

2 garlic cloves, crushed

1 green chilli, deseeded and finely chopped

1 dessertspoon corn oil

2 rounded tablespoons finely chopped fresh coriander

½ teaspoon paprika

black pepper

8 fl.oz/225ml vegetable stock

extra corn oil

Fry the onion, garlic and chilli in the oil until soft. Add the vegetable protein, coriander, paprika and stock and season with black pepper, then stir well and bring to the boil. Cover and simmer, stirring occasionally, for about 5 minutes until the liquid has been absorbed. Remove from the heat and add the mashed beans and breadcrumbs. Mix thoroughly and allow to cool. Take heaped dessertspoonfuls of the mixture and roll into balls. Arrange these in an oiled baking dish and brush each one lightly with oil. Bake in a preheated oven at 180°C/350°F/Gas mark 4 for 25-30 minutes until browned. Serve warm with a salad garnish and salsa.

Avocado and 'cream cheese' spread (serves 4)

1 small avocado, peeled, stoned and chopped

4oz/100g vegan 'cream cheese'

1 tablespoon lemon juice

1 small green chilli, deseeded and finely chopped

1 teaspoon dried parsley

black pepper

Mash the avocado with the lemon juice, then add to the 'cream cheese', chilli and parsley. Season with black pepper and mix until well combined. Use as a spread for tortillas or warm bread.

Canastitas (makes 12)

bases

2oz/50g cornmeal

2oz/50g plain flour

2 tablespoons corn oil

cold water

filling

4oz/100g green pepper, finely chopped

2oz/50g sweetcorn kernels

2oz/50g tomato, skinned and chopped

1 small red onion, peeled and finely chopped

1 small green chilli, deseeded and finely chopped

1 garlic clove, crushed

1 dessertspoon olive oil

1 dessertspoon tomato purée

¼ teaspoon paprika

black pepper

vegan 'Parmesan'

Mix the cornmeal with the flour and stir in the corn oil, then gradually add enough water to bind. Knead the dough well and divide it into 12 equal pieces. Lightly oil a 12-holed small tart tin and roll the pieces of dough out to fit the holes. Prick the bases with a fork and set aside.

Fry the green pepper, onion, chilli and garlic in the olive oil for 5 minutes. Add the sweetcorn, tomato, tomato purée and paprika and season with black pepper. Cook for a couple of minutes while stirring, then divide the filling equally between the bases. Sprinkle the tops with 'Parmesan' and bake in a preheated oven at 180°C/350°F/Gas mark 4 for 15 minutes. Serve warm with a salad garnish.

MAIN COURSES

The main meal of the day can turn into a very lengthy affair, especially when guests are invited and more dishes are prepared. Soup or a selection of appetisers are followed by the main course, which is accompanied by salsas, salads, rice, vegetables and bread or tortillas. A wide variety of dishes, ranging from thick nourishing stews to numerous corn- and other grain-based dishes, are typically enjoyed and most are relatively easy to prepare in spite of the often long list of ingredients.

Vegetable picadillo, variations of which are popular throughout the region, is a very versatile dish and as well as simply being served with rice as a main course it is often used as a filling for tortillas, pancakes or pies or mixed with cooked rice and eaten as a snack.

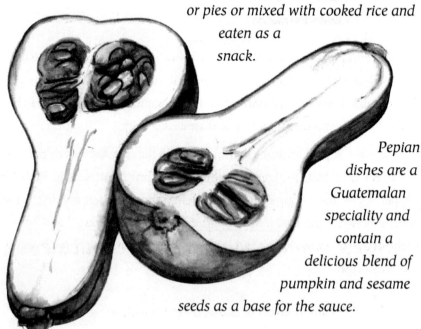

Pepian dishes are a Guatemalan speciality and contain a delicious blend of pumpkin and sesame seeds as a base for the sauce.

Mixed vegetable picadillo (serves 4)

6oz/175g tomatoes, skinned and chopped

4oz/100g courgette, diced

4oz/100g carrots, scraped and diced

4oz/100g red pepper, chopped

4oz/100g green pepper, chopped

4oz/100g mushrooms, wiped and chopped

4oz/100g sweetcorn kernels

2 celery sticks, trimmed and finely chopped

2 garlic cloves, crushed

1 onion, peeled and finely chopped

1 red chilli, deseeded and finely chopped

2oz/50g natural minced textured vegetable protein

1 tablespoon olive oil

1 rounded dessertspoon tomato purée

1 rounded teaspoon dried oregano

1 rounded teaspoon ground cumin

1 teaspoon paprika

12 fl.oz/350ml vegetable stock

black pepper

Heat the oil in a large pan and fry the carrot, celery, garlic, onion and chilli until softened. Add the tomatoes and cook for a couple of minutes, then put in the remaining ingredients. Stir well and bring to the boil, cover and simmer, stirring occasionally, for 15-20 minutes until the mixture is thick and cooked. Serve with plain rice and tortillas.

Sweet potato, banana and peanut stew (serves 4)

1½lb/675g sweet potatoes, peeled and diced

1lb/450g green bananas, peeled and chopped

4oz/100g peanuts, ground and roasted

1 onion, peeled and finely chopped

2 garlic cloves, crushed

1 red chilli, deseeded and finely chopped

1 dessertspoon corn oil

20 fl.oz/600ml vegetable stock

black pepper

roasted chopped peanuts

Fry the onion, garlic and chilli in the oil in a large pan until soft. Add the sweet potato, banana and stock and season with black pepper. Stir well and bring to the boil, then cover and simmer, stirring occasionally, for about 15 minutes until done. Remove from the heat and stir in the ground peanuts. Put back on the stove and bring to the boil again while stirring, then spoon into a serving dish and garnish with chopped peanuts. Serve with a rice dish and wheat tortillas.

Layered garlic rice with savoury mince (serves 4)

12oz/350g long grain rice

4 garlic cloves, crushed

1 tablespoon olive oil

24 fl.oz/725ml water

fresh parsley

filling

6oz/175g tomatoes, skinned and chopped

4oz/100g red pepper, chopped

2oz/50g natural minced textured vegetable protein

1oz/25g raisins

1 onion, peeled and finely chopped

1 garlic clove, crushed

1 small red chilli, deseeded and finely chopped

1 dessertspoon olive oil

1 tablespoon tomato purée

½ teaspoon ground cumin

8 fl.oz/225ml vegetable stock

black pepper

Heat the oil for the filling and fry the onion, garlic, chilli and red pepper for 5 minutes. Add the tomatoes and cook for a few minutes until pulpy, then stir in the remaining filling ingredients. Bring to the boil, cover and simmer, stirring occasionally, for 10 minutes. Uncover and simmer for a few minutes more, stirring frequently, until the liquid has been absorbed. Keep the filling warm while cooking the rice.

Fry the rice and garlic in the oil for 1 minute, then add the water and bring to the boil. Cover and simmer gently until the liquid has been absorbed and the rice is cooked. Oil a deep 8 inch/20cm round loose-bottomed baking tin and spoon one third of the rice into the base. Spread out evenly, then top with half the filling, pressing down firmly. Repeat these layers and finish with the remaining rice. Carefully invert onto a serving plate and lift the tin off. Neaten the edges if necessary and garnish with fresh parsley. Serve with vegetables and bread.

Cornmeal pancakes stuffed with courgette and corn picadillo (serves 4)

pancakes

2oz/50g fine cornmeal

2oz/50g plain flour

1 tablespoon corn oil

10 fl.oz/300ml soya milk

extra corn oil

filling

8oz/225g courgettes, finely diced

8oz/225g sweetcorn kernels

1 onion, peeled and finely chopped

1 green chilli, deseeded and finely chopped

2 garlic cloves, crushed

1 tablespoon corn oil

2 rounded tablespoons finely chopped fresh parsley

1 dessertspoon capers, chopped

black pepper

5 fl.oz/150ml soya milk

1 rounded dessertspoon cornflour

Mix the cornmeal, flour and oil with the soya milk until smooth. Cover and leave to stand for 1 hour. Brush a 7 inch/18cm non-stick frying pan with oil and heat until hot. Whisk the batter again, then put about 2½ tablespoonfuls into the pan. Swirl it around to cover the base of the pan, then cook for a few minutes until golden underneath. Turn the pancake over and cook the other side. Repeat with the remaining batter to make 8 pancakes. Keep them warm while making the filling.

Gently fry the courgette, sweetcorn, onion, chilli and garlic in the oil, stirring frequently, for 15 minutes. Mix the cornflour with the soya milk until smooth and add to the pan together with the parsley and capers. Season with black pepper and bring to the boil while stirring. Continue stirring for a minute or so until the mixture thickens.

Divide the filling between the warm pancakes, folding or rolling each one up to enclose it. Serve with a salsa and salad.

Aubergine and kidney bean salsa stew (serves 4)

1½lb/675g aubergines, diced

8oz/225g cooked red kidney beans

1 onion, peeled and finely chopped

4 tablespoons olive oil

1 quantity tomato and chilli salsa (see page 84)

finely chopped fresh coriander

Fry the aubergine and onion in the oil in a large pan for 10 minutes, stirring frequently to prevent sticking. Add the salsa and simmer for 5 minutes, then put in the beans and continue simmering, stirring frequently, for a further 5 minutes until the mixture is cooked and thick. Garnish with chopped coriander and serve with a rice dish and warm bread.

Pepper and bean flan (serves 4)

base

3oz/75g cornmeal

3oz/75g plain flour

1 teaspoon baking powder

2oz/50g vegan margarine

cold water

filling

8oz/225g mixed peppers, chopped

6oz/175g cooked mixed beans

6oz/175g tomatoes, skinned and chopped

1 red onion, peeled and finely chopped

2 garlic cloves, crushed

1 small red chilli, deseeded and finely chopped

1 tablespoon olive oil

1 dessertspoon tomato purée

½ teaspoon paprika

½ teaspoon dried thyme

black pepper

chopped walnuts

grated vegan 'cheese' (optional)

Mix the cornmeal with the sifted flour and baking powder and rub in the margarine. Add enough water to bind, then knead the dough well and turn it out onto a floured board. Roll out to line a greased deep loose-bottomed 8 inch/20cm diameter flan tin. Prick the base all over with a fork and bake blind in a preheated oven at 180°C/350°F/Gas mark 4 for 10 minutes.

Heat the oil in a large pan and fry the peppers, onion, garlic and chilli for 5 minutes, stirring frequently. Add the tomatoes, beans, tomato purée, paprika and thyme and season with black pepper. Raise the heat and simmer, stirring frequently, for 5 minutes. Spoon the filling evenly into the flan case, return it to the oven and bake for 25 minutes. Carefully remove the flan from the tin and sprinkle walnuts and if liked grated 'cheese' on top. Cut into 4 wedges and serve with vegetable and salad accompaniments.

Baked dumpling gratin (serves 4)

> 4 steamed corn dumplings (see page 65)
> 12oz/350g tomatoes, skinned and chopped
> 4oz/100g green pepper, chopped
> 4oz/100g red pepper, chopped
> 1 onion, peeled and finely chopped
> 2 garlic cloves, crushed
> 1 green chilli, deseeded and finely chopped
> 1 tablespoon olive oil
> 2 fl.oz/50ml water
> 1 rounded dessertspoon tomato purée
> ½ teaspoon paprika
> black pepper
> 1½oz/40g breadcrumbs
> 1 rounded dessertspoon vegan 'Parmesan'

Fry the green and red peppers, onion, garlic and chilli in the oil for a few minutes to soften. Add the tomatoes, water, tomato purée and paprika and season with black pepper, stir well and bring to the boil. Cover and simmer, stirring occasionally, for 5 minutes. Meanwhile chop the cooked dumplings and put them in a greased casserole dish. Spoon the sauce evenly over the top, then mix the breadcrumbs with the 'Parmesan' and sprinkle over the sauce. Cover and bake in a preheated oven at 180°C/350°F/Gas mark 4 for 30 minutes. Uncover and bake for another 5 minutes until golden brown. Serve with vegetables and salad.

Roasted pepper, chickpea and sweetcorn pepian (serves 4)

1lb/450g mixed peppers

8oz/225g cooked chickpeas

8oz/225g sweetcorn kernels

4oz/100g pumpkin seeds

2 rounded tablespoons sesame seeds

8oz/225g tomatoes, skinned and chopped

1 onion, peeled and chopped

4 garlic cloves, chopped

1-2 green chillies, deseeded and chopped

2 tablespoons corn oil

2 rounded tablespoons finely chopped fresh parsley

½ teaspoon ground allspice

black pepper

10 fl.oz/300ml vegetable stock

extra pumpkin seeds

Roast the peppers under a hot grill until the skins blister. Allow to cool slightly, then remove the skins, stalks, membranes and seeds and chop the flesh. Roast the pumpkin and sesame seeds until lightly golden and grind them finely. Blend the tomatoes, onion, garlic and chillies to a purée, add the ground seeds, parsley and allspice, season with black pepper and mix to a thick paste. Heat the oil in a large pan and fry the paste, stirring constantly, for 5 minutes. Remove from the heat and add the chopped peppers, chickpeas, sweetcorn and stock and mix thoroughly. Return to the heat, bring to the boil, cover and simmer for 10 minutes, stirring frequently. Transfer to a serving dish and sprinkle with pumpkin seeds. Serve with a rice dish and bread.

Quinoa with mixed vegetables (serves 4)

8oz/225g quinoa

16 fl.oz/475ml water

8oz/225g potatoes, peeled and finely diced

8oz/225g carrots, scraped and finely diced

8oz/225g chayotes, peeled and finely diced

6oz/175g sweetcorn kernels

6oz/175g cooked red kidney beans

1 onion, peeled and chopped

1 red chilli, deseeded and finely chopped

2 garlic cloves, crushed

1 dessertspoon corn oil

14oz/400g tin crushed tomatoes

20 fl.oz/600ml vegetable stock

1 tablespoon tomato purée

2 teaspoons ground cumin

¼ teaspoon ground allspice

black pepper

grated vegan 'cheese'

chopped pecans

Put the quinoa and water in a saucepan and bring to the boil. Cover and simmer for about 15 minutes until the liquid has been absorbed, then remove from the heat. Fry the onion, chilli and garlic in the oil in a large pan until softened. Add the potato, carrot, chayote and stock and bring to the boil. Cover and simmer for 15 minutes. Remove from the heat and add the crushed tomatoes, sweetcorn, kidney beans, tomato purée, cumin, allspice and quinoa. Season with black pepper and mix well. Put back on the cooker and bring to the boil. Simmer for 5 minutes, stirring frequently, then spoon into a serving dish and garnish with grated 'cheese' and chopped pecans. Serve with warm cornbread and a salad.

Green chilli and potato stew (serves 4)

1¼lb/550g potatoes, peeled and diced

1lb/450g green peppers, sliced

1lb/450g tomatoes, skinned and chopped

1 onion, peeled and sliced

2 green chillies, deseeded and finely chopped

2 garlic cloves, crushed

1 dessertspoon olive oil

1 tablespoon tomato purée

16 fl.oz/475ml vegetable stock

black pepper

2 fl.oz/50ml water

1oz/25g cornflour

green chilli rings

Heat the oil in a large pan and fry the onion, garlic and chopped chillies for 5 minutes. Add the potatoes, green peppers, tomatoes, tomato purée and vegetable stock and season with black pepper. Stir well and bring to the boil. Cover and simmer, stirring occasionally, for about 30 minutes until the potatoes are done. Mix the cornflour with the water until smooth and add to the pan. Continue simmering while stirring for a minute or two until the stew thickens. Garnish with chilli rings and serve with a rice dish and warm bread.

Layered wheat tortilla pie (serves 4)

6 7inch/18cm wheat tortillas (see page 90)

shredded lettuce

filling

8oz/225g cooked spinach, finely chopped

8oz/225g courgettes, finely chopped

1 onion, peeled and finely chopped

1 green chilli, deseeded and finely chopped

2 garlic cloves, crushed

1 tablespoon corn oil

2oz/50g vegan 'cheese', grated

4 fl.oz/125ml soya milk

1 rounded dessertspoon cornflour

1 teaspoon dried thyme

black pepper

Fry the courgette, onion, chilli and garlic in the oil in a large pan for 10 minutes. Add the spinach and thyme and season with black pepper, stirring around until well combined. Mix the cornflour with the soya milk until smooth, then add to the pan together with the grated 'cheese'. Bring to the boil while stirring and continue stirring for a minute or so until the mixture thickens. Put a wheat tortilla in a deep 7 inch/18cm ramekin dish and cover with a layer of filling. Repeat these layers four times and finish with the remaining tortilla. Press down firmly and evenly, then cover with foil and bake in a preheated oven at 180°C/350°F/Gas mark 4 for 30 minutes. Run a sharp knife around the edges to loosen and invert the pie onto a serving plate. Arrange some shredded lettuce around the edge and cut the pie into wedges with a sharp knife. Serve with a salsa and rice accompaniment.

Corn-topped aubergine and savoury mince pie (serves 4)

1lb/450g aubergines, finely diced

8oz/225g tomatoes, skinned and chopped

2oz/50g natural minced textured vegetable protein

1oz/25g raisins

1 red onion, peeled and finely chopped

1 red chilli, deseeded and finely chopped

2 garlic cloves, crushed

3 tablespoons corn oil

1 tablespoon tomato purée

1 teaspoon ground cumin

½ teaspoon paprika

black pepper

12 fl.oz/350ml vegetable stock

topping

4oz/100g sweetcorn kernels

4oz/100g cornmeal

2oz/50g plain flour

1oz/25g vegan margarine, melted

1 small onion, peeled and grated

1 teaspoon baking powder

¼ teaspoon cayenne pepper

In a large pan, fry the aubergine, onion, garlic and chilli in the oil for 10 minutes, stirring frequently. Add the tomatoes, vegetable protein, raisins, tomato purée, cumin, paprika and stock and season with black pepper. Stir well and bring to the boil. Cover and simmer gently, stirring occasionally, for 10 minutes. Spoon the mixture evenly into a 10 x 7 inch/25 x 18cm greased baking dish.

Blanch the sweetcorn, then drain over a bowl and blend with 4 fl.oz/125ml of its cooking liquid. Transfer to a mixing bowl and stir in the margarine and onion. Add the cornmeal, sifted flour and baking powder and cayenne pepper and combine well. Spoon the mixture evenly over the base in the baking dish and bake in a preheated oven at 180°C/350°F/Gas mark 4 for about 35 minutes until golden. Serve with a vegetable or salad.

Red pepian, sweet potato and paw paw stew (serves 4)

1lb/450g sweet potatoes, peeled and diced

1 underripe paw paw, peeled, deseeded and diced

8oz/225g red peppers, chopped

8oz/225g tomatoes, skinned and chopped

2 garlic cloves, crushed

1-2 red chillies, deseeded and chopped

1 red onion, peeled and finely chopped

2oz/50g pumpkin seeds, roasted and ground

1 rounded tablespoon sesame seeds, roasted and ground

1 tablespoon tomato purée

1 tablespoon corn oil

1 rounded tablespoon finely chopped fresh coriander

14 fl.oz/425ml vegetable stock

½ teaspoon paprika

black pepper

extra roasted sesame seeds

Blend the tomatoes with the garlic and chillies until smooth, then put in a bowl and add the ground pumpkin and sesame seeds, tomato purée and paprika. Mix to a paste. Heat the oil in a large pan and fry the onion until softened. Add the paste and while stirring fry for 5 minutes. Remove from the stove and add the potato, paw paw, red pepper, coriander and stock and season with black pepper. Stir well and return to the heat. Bring to the boil, then cover and simmer, stirring frequently, for about 25 minutes until tender. Transfer to a serving bowl and sprinkle with roasted sesame seeds. Serve with a rice dish and warm bread.

Butternut squash and cornmeal pie (serves 4)

2lb/900g butternut squash, peeled, deseeded and diced

6oz/175g tomatoes, skinned and chopped

6oz/175g cooked red kidney beans

4oz/100g red pepper, finely chopped

1 red onion, peeled and finely chopped

2 garlic cloves, crushed

8 fl.oz/225ml vegetable stock

1 dessertspoon corn oil

1 rounded teaspoon ground cumin

¼ teaspoon cayenne pepper

black pepper

topping

4oz/100g cornmeal

20 fl.oz/600ml vegetable stock

Fry the red pepper, onion and garlic in the oil for 3 minutes, then add the tomato, cumin and cayenne pepper and cook for 2 minutes. Add the squash and 8 fl.oz/225ml of stock, season with black pepper, stir well and bring to the boil. Cover and simmer, stirring occasionally, for 15-20 minutes until cooked and thick. Remove from the heat and stir in the beans.

Put the 20 fl.oz/600ml of stock in a large pan and bring to the boil. Remove from the heat and gradually add the cornmeal, whisking all the time until smooth and without lumps. Return to a low heat and cook, stirring frequently, for 10 minutes, but be careful not to turn up the heat too high as the mixture tends to spit out if this happens. Spoon the vegetable mixture into a greased deep casserole dish of about 10 x 9 inches/25 x 23cm and spread the cornmeal evenly on top. Bake in a preheated oven at 180°C/350°F/Gas mark 4 for about 35 minutes until golden brown. Serve with vegetable or salad accompaniments.

ACCOMPANIMENTS

Frijoles, beans, are such a fundamental staple that there is invariably a large pot simmering away on the stove in Central American households. Cooked beans are used in countless recipes or just served as an accompaniment to other dishes. Refried beans are simply mashed beans fried with onion and garlic, which are then used as a topping or filling and in numerous other recipes.

As well as the other typical accompaniments featured here, plantains cooked in various ways are also extremely popular. These are commonly peeled and sliced lengthways and fried until golden, or steamed or boiled until tender, mashed and shaped into balls. Cassava, an important staple root vegetable grown all over the region, is treated in the same way as a potato and served boiled, mashed, baked or fried.

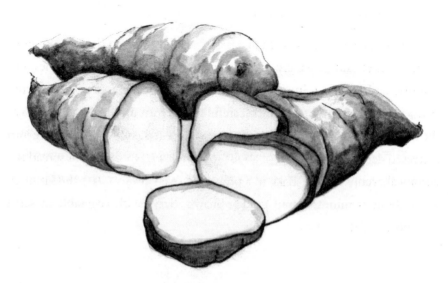

Frijoles

Black beans

1lb/450g dried black beans

4 garlic cloves, chopped

few sprigs of fresh coriander

Pinto or red kidney beans

1lb/450g dried pinto or red kidney beans

1 tablespoon tomato purée

4 garlic cloves, crushed

1 red chilli, chopped

Soak the beans in water overnight, drain and rinse and put in a pan of fresh water. Bring to the boil, then drain and rinse again, cover with fresh water and add the remaining ingredients for either black or pinto/red beans. Bring to the boil, cover and simmer for 1¼-1½ hours until the beans are soft. Drain and keep the cooking liquid for stock.

Refried beans

8oz/225g cooked black, pinto or red kidney beans

1 small onion, peeled and finely chopped

2 garlic cloves crushed

1 tablespoon corn oil

Soften the onion and garlic in the oil. Remove from the heat, add the beans and mash smooth. Return to the stove and cook, stirring continuously, for 5 minutes. Serve as an accompaniment or use as a topping for breads or tortillas. Refried beans can also be thinned with a little water and served as a dip.

Spiced mixed beans (serves 4)

8oz/225g cooked mixed beans

8oz/225g tomatoes, skinned and chopped

4oz/100g carrots, scraped and finely chopped

1 red onion, peeled and finely chopped

1 red chilli, deseeded and finely chopped

1 garlic clove, crushed

1 tablespoon corn oil

1 rounded dessertspoon tomato purée

1 rounded teaspoon ground cumin

¼ teaspoon ground allspice

black pepper

finely chopped fresh coriander

Fry the carrot, onion, chilli and garlic in the oil for 5 minutes, then add the ground cumin and allspice and stir around for a few seconds. Add the tomatoes and tomato purée and cook for a couple of minutes. Put in the beans and season with black pepper. Simmer for a few minutes, adding a little water if necessary to prevent sticking, and stir until the mixture is thick. Transfer to a serving bowl and sprinkle with chopped coriander.

Spinach with black beans (serves 4)

12oz/350g fresh spinach, shredded

8oz/225g cooked black beans

1 onion, peeled and finely chopped

1 green chilli, deseeded and finely chopped

1 garlic clove, crushed

1 dessertspoon corn oil

1 teaspoon dried thyme

black pepper

Heat the oil in a large pan and fry the onion, chilli and garlic until soft. Add the spinach and cook for about 5 minutes until it wilts. Stir in the beans and thyme and season with black pepper, adding a little water if necessary to prevent sticking. Cook for 2-3 minutes more until the spinach is tender.

Sweet potato and squash purée (serves 4)

12oz/350g sweet potatoes, peeled

12oz/350g butternut squash, peeled

1 onion, peeled and finely chopped

1 dessertspoon corn oil

1 teaspoon ground cumin

¼ teaspoon cayenne pepper

black pepper

Fry the onion in the oil until soft. Meanwhile cut the sweet potatoes and squash into even-sized pieces and steam until done. Add the cumin and cayenne pepper to the onion and stir around briefly. Now add the cooked potato and squash, season with black pepper and mash until smooth and well combined. Serve immediately, or alternatively transfer to a baking dish, cover and warm in a moderate oven before serving.

Broccoli with avocado sauce (serves 4)

1lb/450g broccoli, chopped

1 medium avocado, peeled, stoned and mashed

1 onion, peeled and chopped

1 green chilli, deseeded and finely chopped

2 garlic cloves, crushed

1 dessertspoon corn oil

1 teaspoon dried thyme

black pepper

8 fl.oz/225ml vegetable stock

5 fl.oz/150ml soya milk

1 rounded dessertspoon cornflour

finely chopped fresh parsley

Fry the onion, chilli and garlic in the oil until softened. Add the broccoli, thyme and vegetable stock and season with black pepper. Stir well and bring to the boil, then cover and simmer for about 10 minutes, stirring occasionally, until cooked. Mix the cornflour with the soya milk until smooth and add to the pan together with the mashed avocado. Combine well and bring to the boil while stirring. Continue stirring for a minute or so until the sauce thickens, then spoon into a serving dish and sprinkle with chopped parsley.

Creamed corn (serves 4)

1lb/450g sweetcorn kernels

6 fl.oz/175ml coconut milk

1 onion, peeled and finely chopped

1 small green chilli, deseeded and finely chopped

1 dessertspoon corn oil

black pepper

finely chopped fresh coriander

Blanch the sweetcorn kernels if fresh or frozen, then drain and blend with the coconut milk. Fry the onion and chilli in the oil until soft and add the blended corn. Season with black pepper and cook while stirring for about 3 minutes until thick. Serve sprinkled with coriander.

Baked marinated courgettes (serves 4)

1½lb/675g courgettes, halved lengthways and sliced

   marinade

6oz/175g tomatoes, skinned and chopped

2 garlic cloves, crushed

2 rounded tablespoons finely chopped fresh coriander

1 tablespoon lime juice

1 tablespoon tomato purée

1 tablespoon olive oil

dash of Tabasco sauce

black pepper

Blend all the marinade ingredients together until smooth and pour into a large bowl. Add the courgettes, mix well, cover and leave to marinate in the fridge for a few hours. Transfer to a baking dish, cover and bake in a preheated oven at 180°C/350°F/Gas mark 4 for 35-40 minutes until tender.

Chayotes maria (serves 4)

1¼lb/550g chayotes, peeled

8 fl.oz/225ml soya milk

2 rounded tablespoons finely chopped fresh parsley

1 garlic clove, crushed

3 spring onions, trimmed and finely sliced

1 dessertspoon corn oil

1 rounded tablespoon cornflour

black pepper

Cook the chayotes. Meanwhile fry the garlic and spring onions in the oil. Mix the cornflour with the soya milk until smooth and add to the onion and garlic, together with the parsley. Season with black pepper and stir well. Bring to the boil while stirring and continue stirring for a minute or so until the sauce thickens. Drain the cooked chayotes and cut them into slices, removing the inner stones. Put them in a serving dish and pour the hot sauce over the top.

Corn with tomato and green pepper (serves 4)

6oz/175g sweetcorn kernels

6oz/175g tomatoes, skinned and chopped

6oz/175g green peppers, chopped

1 onion, peeled and finely chopped

2 garlic cloves, crushed

1 tablespoon olive oil

1 dessertspoon capers, chopped

½ teaspoon dried oregano

¼ teaspoon cayenne pepper

black pepper

grated vegan 'cheese'

Fry the green pepper, onion and garlic in the oil until softened. Add the remaining ingredients except the 'cheese' and simmer, stirring occasionally, for 10 minutes. Spoon into a dish and garnish with grated 'cheese'.

Green vegetables with quinoa (serves 4)

4oz/100g broccoli, chopped

4oz/100g courgette, diced

4oz/100g green beans, topped, tailed and cut into ½ inch/1cm lengths

4oz/100g quinoa

1 onion, peeled and finely chopped

1 green chilli, deseeded and finely chopped

1 garlic clove, crushed

1 dessertspoon corn oil

12 fl.oz/350ml vegetable stock

1 teaspoon dried oregano

black pepper

finely chopped fresh parsley

Soften the onion, chilli and garlic in the oil. Add the remaining ingredients apart from the parsley and stir well, then bring to the boil, cover and simmer gently until the liquid has been absorbed. Garnish with chopped parsley before serving.

Spiced courgettes with amaranth (serves 4)

12oz/350g courgettes, chopped

4oz/100g amaranth

1 onion, peeled and finely chopped

1 green chilli, deseeded and finely chopped

1 garlic clove, crushed

1 tablespoon corn oil

1 teaspoon ground coriander

1 teaspoon ground cumin

¼ teaspoon ground allspice

black pepper

10 fl.oz/300ml vegetable stock

finely chopped fresh coriander

Bring the amaranth and stock to the boil, cover and simmer gently for about 20 minutes until the liquid has been absorbed. Meanwhile fry the onion in the oil for 3 minutes, then put in the courgettes, chilli and garlic and continue cooking, stirring frequently, until just tender. Add the ground coriander, cumin and allspice and stir around for 30 seconds. Remove from the heat and add the cooked amaranth, then season with black pepper and mix until well combined. Transfer to a serving dish and garnish with chopped coriander.

SNACKS

Savoury little pies and flans and stuffed pancakes, fritters and dumplings are typical of the type of snack foods that can be bought ready-made from street vendors at all times of the day. These little snacks are also commonly made at home, often using leftovers from other meals.

Steamed corn dumplings are a favourite in Guatemala and are traditionally steamed in the papery husks that surround corncobs. Corn-on-the-cob too, naturally, makes a very popular snack and is served roasted, boiled, baked, steamed or barbecued. Stuffed chayotes are also a speciality and these are simply boiled until tender, then cut in half, hollowed out and filled with a savoury filling such as picadillo, a salsa or 'cream cheese'.

To make more of a meal of any of these snacks they can be served with a rice dish and salad accompaniments.

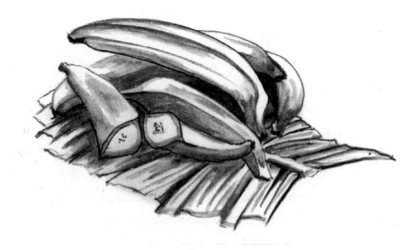

Pupusas (makes 8)

pastry

4oz/100g plain flour

2oz/50g cornmeal

2oz/50g vegan margarine

cold water

filling

4oz/100g carrots, scraped and grated

2oz/50g cooked red kidney beans, mashed

2oz/50g tomato, skinned and chopped

1oz/25g natural minced textured vegetable protein

1 small red onion, peeled and finely chopped

1 garlic clove, crushed

1 red chilli, deseeded and finely chopped

1 dessertspoon corn oil

¼ teaspoon paprika

black pepper

4 fl.oz/125ml vegetable stock

1oz/25g vegan 'cheese', grated

Fry the carrot, onion, garlic and chilli in the oil until softened. Add the tomato, vegetable protein, paprika and stock and season with black pepper. Stir well and bring to the boil, cover and simmer for 5 minutes. Remove from the heat and stir in the mashed beans, then set aside to cool.

Mix the flour with the cornmeal and rub in the margarine. Add enough water to make a soft dough, then turn this out onto a floured board and knead well. Divide the dough into 8 equal pieces and roll each one out on a floured board into a circle of about 5 inches/13cm. Divide the cooled filling between the pastry circles, placing it neatly on one half of each circle. Sprinkle the grated 'cheese' over the filling and dampen the pastry edges with water. Fold the pastry over to enclose the filling and pinch the edges together to join. Brush a non-stick frying pan with oil and heat until hot. Fry the pupusas for a few minutes on each side until golden brown, then serve hot.

Plantain fritters (makes 8)

12oz/350g yellow plantains, peeled and chopped

1 onion, peeled and grated

1 garlic clove, crushed

1oz/25g plain flour

¼ teaspoon cayenne pepper

black pepper

water

corn oil

Steam the plantain until done, then mash and add the onion, garlic, flour and cayenne pepper. Season with black pepper and combine well. Add a little water to bind, then take rounded tablespoonfuls of the mixture and roll into balls in the palm of the hand. Flatten the balls and shallow fry them for a few minutes on each side until browned. Drain on kitchen paper and serve warm.

Sweetcorn torte (serves 4)

8oz/225g sweetcorn kernels

4oz/100g cornmeal

1oz/25g vegan 'cheese', grated

1oz/25g vegan margarine

1 onion, peeled and finely chopped

1 red chilli, deseeded and finely chopped

1 garlic clove, crushed

black pepper

Cook the sweetcorn, drain over a bowl and keep 4 fl.oz/125ml of the cooking liquid. Blend half of the sweetcorn with this liquid, then stir it into the remaining sweetcorn.

Fry the onion, chilli and garlic in the margarine until soft, remove from the heat and add the sweetcorn, cornmeal and 'cheese'. Season with black pepper and mix thoroughly. Spoon the mixture into a greased 7 inch/18cm round loose-bottomed flan tin and level the top. Bake in a preheated oven at 180°C/350°F/Gas mark 4 for about 30 minutes until golden and set. Run a knife around the edges to loosen and carefully remove the torte from the tin. Cut into wedges and serve warm, topped with a salsa.

Baked stuffed tortillas (serves 4)

4 7inch/18cm wheat tortillas (see page 90)

corn oil

sesame seeds

filling

12oz/350g aubergine, finely chopped

1 red onion, peeled and finely chopped

1 small red chilli, deseeded and finely chopped

2 garlic cloves, crushed

2 tablespoons corn oil

1oz/25g natural minced textured vegetable protein

dash of Tabasco sauce

¼ teaspoon ground allspice

1 rounded teaspoon ground cumin

black pepper

7 fl.oz/200ml vegetable stock

Heat the oil and fry the aubergine, onion, chilli and garlic for 10 minutes, stirring frequently. Add the remaining filling ingredients and combine well. Bring to the boil, then cover and simmer for 5 minutes. Uncover and simmer for a further 5 minutes or so, stirring occasionally, until the liquid has been absorbed and the mixture is thick. Meanwhile, heat the tortillas briefly in a warm oven to soften them. Divide the filling equally between the tortillas, putting it on one half of each one only. Fold each tortilla over to enclose the filling, then arrange them in a greased baking dish. Brush the tops with oil and sprinkle with sesame seeds. Bake in a preheated oven at 180°C/350°F/Gas mark 4 for 10-15 minutes until golden brown. Serve hot.

Picadillo pies (makes 4)

pastry
2oz/50g cornmeal
2oz/50g plain flour
1 teaspoon baking powder
2 tablespoons corn oil
cold water
filling
¼ quantity vegetable picadillo (see page 37)
grated vegan 'cheese'

Put the cornmeal and sifted flour and baking powder in a mixing bowl and stir in the oil. Gradually add enough water to bind, then knead the dough and divide it into 4 equal portions. Roll each one into a ball, then flatten them into rounds to line 4 individual greased 4 inch/10cm round flan tins. Prick the bases and bake blind in a preheated oven at 180°C/350°F/Gas mark 4 for 15 minutes.

Heat the picadillo and divide it equally between the flan cases. Return to the oven for 10 minutes, then carefully remove the flans from the tins and sprinkle the grated 'cheese' on top. Serve hot.

Stuffed cassava fritters (makes 8)

1½lb/675g cassava, peeled
½ quantity refried beans (see page 51)
corn oil

Cut the cassava into even-sized chunks and cook them. Drain and mash the cassava, then divide it into 8 equal portions. Roll each one into a ball, then shape these into small cups. Fill them with refried beans and push the top of the cups over to seal and enclose the filling. Put the filled balls on a flat surface and shape them into ovals of about ½ inch/1cm thick. Shallow fry the fritters in hot oil for a few minutes on each side until golden. Drain on kitchen paper and serve hot.

Panamanian empanadas (makes 6)

pastry

6oz/175g plain flour

1 rounded teaspoon baking powder

2oz/50g vegan margarine

cold water

filling

4oz/100g red pepper, finely chopped

2oz/50g tomato, skinned and chopped

1oz/25g natural minced textured vegetable protein

½oz/15g raisins

1 onion, peeled and finely chopped

1 garlic clove, crushed

1 red chilli, deseeded and finely chopped

5 fl.oz/150ml vegetable stock

1 dessertspoon corn oil

1 teaspoon dried thyme

¼ teaspoon ground allspice

black pepper

Fry the red pepper, onion, garlic and chilli in the oil for 5 minutes. Add the remaining filling ingredients and stir well, then bring to the boil, cover and simmer for 5 minutes. Uncover and simmer for another 5 minutes or so, stirring regularly, until the liquid has been absorbed. Remove from the heat and allow to cool.

Rub the margarine into the sifted flour and baking powder in a mixing bowl. Add enough water to bind, then knead the dough well and divide it into 6 equal portions. Roll each one into a ball and then into a 6 inch/15cm circle on a floured board. Divide the filling between the circles, placing it on one side only. Dampen the pastry edges with water and fold over to enclose the filling. Roll the edges together to join and make a couple of slits in the top of each empanada with a sharp knife. Transfer to a greased baking sheet and bake in a preheated oven at 180°C/350°F/Gas mark 4 for about 25 minutes until golden brown. Serve hot.

Potato and onion pancake (serves 4)

12oz/350g potatoes, peeled

1 onion, peeled and finely chopped

2 garlic cloves, crushed

1 dessertspoon olive oil

2oz/50g cornmeal

2oz/50g plain flour

1 teaspoon baking powder

8 fl.oz/225ml soya milk

black pepper

Mix the cornmeal with the sifted flour and baking powder, black pepper and soya milk until smooth, then cover and set aside. Boil the potato, drain and allow to cool, then finely chop it. Fry the onion and garlic in the oil in a 9 inch/23cm non-stick frying pan until soft. Add the potato and stir around for 1 minute. Remove the pan from the heat to add the batter, mixing it well with the potato and onion, then cook over a medium heat for about 10 minutes until the underside is browned. Now put the frying pan under a medium hot grill for about 10 minutes until the top is golden brown and the pancake is set. Carefully transfer to a serving plate and cut into 4 wedges. Serve hot.

Steamed corn dumplings (makes 4)

dough

4oz/100g sweetcorn kernels, cooked

2 fl.oz/50ml vegetable stock

3oz/75g cornmeal

3oz/75g plain flour

1 rounded teaspoon baking powder

filling

4oz/100g cooked pinto or black beans, mashed

1oz/25g vegan 'cheese', grated

1 small onion, peeled and finely chopped

2 garlic cloves, crushed

1 dessertspoon corn oil

1 teaspoon dried thyme

¼ teaspoon cayenne pepper

black pepper

Heat the oil and fry the onion and garlic until soft, then remove from the heat, add the remaining filling ingredients and combine well.

Blend the sweetcorn kernels with the vegetable stock, then transfer to a large bowl and add the cornmeal and sifted flour and baking powder. Mix thoroughly until a soft dough forms. Turn this out onto a floured board and divide it into 4 equal portions. Roll each piece in flour and then into a ball in the palm of the hand. Flatten these into 4 inch/10cm circles and spoon a quarter of the filling in the centre of each one. Re-form the dough into balls, pinching the edges together to join and to enclose the filling. Wrap the dumplings individually in foil and place them in a steamer. Steam for 25 minutes, then serve hot.

Bean-filled plantain pancakes (serves 4)

12oz/350g yellow plantains, peeled and chopped

⅓ quantity refried beans (see page 51)

8 fl.oz/225ml vegetable stock

1 dessertspoon lemon juice

3oz/75g plain flour

½oz/15g vegan margarine

black pepper

extra flour

corn oil

Put the plantain, lemon juice and stock in a saucepan and bring to the boil. Cover and simmer, stirring occasionally, for about 20 minutes until tender. Add the margarine and stir around until melted, then remove from the heat and mash the plantains. Season with black pepper, add the flour and mix thoroughly. Divide both the plantain mixture and the refried beans into 8 equal portions. Take one portion of plantain mixture and roll it into a ball with dampened hands, then form this into a cup and fill with a portion of refried beans. Fold the plantain over to enclose the filling, dip lightly in flour and flatten into an oval pancake. Repeat with the remaining portions. Shallow fry the pancakes in hot oil for a few minutes on each side until golden. Drain on kitchen paper and serve hot.

RICE

Since it was first introduced by the Spanish in the 16th century, rice has become a major agricultural crop and a staple food throughout the region. Rice and beans, gallo pinto, is ubiquitous and considered to be a national dish in many of the countries. Although variations are found in different countries, the dish is very often served as a complete meal and is typically accompanied by cabbage salad, fried plantains and chopped avocado. In many poorer areas rice and beans is the subsistence food and is eaten at every mealtime. From a nutritional point of view rice and beans offer a perfect combination of amino acids, so, eaten together, they provide a complete source of protein.

Long grain white is the most widely used variety and when served plain it is invariably cooked in the cooking liquid from beans. Any leftover rice is commonly fried and used for the next meal or added to other ingredients and used as a filling or topping for tortillas.

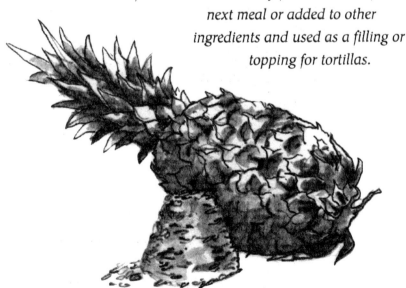

Gallo pinto (serves 4)

8oz/225g long grain rice

8oz/225g cooked black or pinto beans

1 onion, peeled and finely chopped

2 garlic cloves, crushed

2 tablespoons olive oil

2 rounded tablespoons finely chopped fresh coriander

dash of Tabasco sauce

black pepper

1 small avocado, peeled, stoned and chopped

Cook the rice, then drain and rinse and refrigerate for a few hours until cold. Heat the oil in a pan and fry the onion and garlic until soft. Add the cooked rice and beans, coriander and Tabasco sauce and season with black pepper. Fry while stirring for 5 minutes, then transfer to a serving dish and garnish with chopped avocado.

Guatemalan vegetable rice (serves 4)

8oz/225g long grain rice

8oz/225g prepared vegetables (e.g. a mixture of celery, carrots, peppers, peas and sweetcorn), finely chopped as necessary

1 tablespoon olive oil

18 fl.oz/525ml vegetable stock

black pepper

finely chopped fresh parsley

Fry the rice in the olive oil for a few minutes. Add the vegetables and stock and season with black pepper, then bring to the boil, cover and simmer gently until the liquid has been absorbed. Spoon into a serving dish and sprinkle with chopped parsley.

Tomato and 'cheese' rice (serves 4)

8oz/225g long grain rice

8oz/225g tomatoes, skinned and chopped

4oz/100g green pepper, chopped

1 red onion, peeled and finely chopped

1 dessertspoon olive oil

1 dessertspoon tomato purée

dash of Tabasco sauce

black pepper

16 fl.oz/475ml vegetable stock

2oz/50g vegan 'cheese', grated

chopped green olives

finely chopped fresh parsley

Soften the onion in the oil. Add the tomato and green pepper and cook for a couple of minutes to soften, then stir in the rice, tomato purée, Tabasco sauce and stock and season with black pepper. Bring to the boil, cover and simmer gently until the liquid has been absorbed. Remove from the heat and stir in the grated 'cheese'. Serve garnished with chopped olives and parsley.

Picadillo rice (serves 4)

¼ quantity mixed vegetable picadillo (see page 37)

6oz/175g long grain rice

chopped walnuts

finely chopped fresh parsley

Gently heat the picadillo in a pan until hot. Cook the rice, then drain and rinse with boiling water. Drain well and mix with the hot picadillo. Spoon into a serving dish and sprinkle with chopped walnuts and parsley.

Coconut rice with beans (serves 4)

8oz/225g long grain rice

8oz/225g cooked red kidney beans

8oz/225g green peppers, chopped

1 onion, peeled and finely chopped

2 garlic cloves, crushed

1 tablespoon corn oil

1 teaspoon dried thyme

black pepper

20 fl.oz/600ml vegetable stock

1oz/25g creamed coconut, grated

finely chopped fresh coriander

Fry the green pepper, onion and garlic in the oil until softened. Add the rice, kidney beans, thyme and stock and season with black pepper. Stir well and bring to the boil, cover and simmer gently until the liquid has been absorbed. Remove from the heat and stir in the coconut. Garnish with chopped coriander before serving.

Rice moulds with hearts of palm (serves 4)

8oz/225g long grain rice

14oz/400g tin hearts of palm, drained, rinsed and finely chopped

1 onion, peeled and finely chopped

1 garlic clove, crushed

1 dessertspoon olive oil

18 fl.oz/525ml vegetable stock

2 fl.oz/50ml white wine

black pepper

1oz/25g vegan 'cheese', grated

fresh parsley sprigs

Heat the oil and fry the onion and garlic until soft. Add the rice, hearts of palm, stock and wine and season with black pepper, stir well and bring to the boil. Cover and simmer gently until the liquid has been absorbed. Remove from the heat and stir in the 'cheese'. Lightly oil 4 small ramekins dishes and divide the rice between them, pressing it down firmly. Refrigerate for a few hours, then run a sharp knife around the edges to loosen and carefully invert the rice moulds onto plates. Garnish each mould with a sprig of parsley.

Pineapple rice (serves 4)

8oz/225g long grain rice

8oz/225g tin pineapple chunks in natural juice

1oz/25g raisins

1 onion, peeled and finely chopped

1 dessertspoon corn oil

16 fl.oz/475ml vegetable stock

¼ teaspoon turmeric

black pepper

grated creamed coconut

finely chopped fresh coriander

Fry the onion in the oil until soft. Add the rice and turmeric and stir around for a few seconds. Chop the pineapple into smaller pieces and add to the pan together with the juice, raisins and stock. Season with black pepper and stir well. Bring to the boil, then cover and simmer gently until the liquid has been absorbed. Transfer to a serving dish and sprinkle with grated creamed coconut and fresh coriander.

Fried spiced rice (serves 4)

8oz/225g long grain rice

1 onion, peeled and finely chopped

2 garlic cloves, crushed

1 green chilli, deseeded and finely chopped

1oz/25g raisins

2 tablespoons corn oil

1 teaspoon ground coriander

1 teaspoon ground cumin

½ teaspoon ground allspice

black pepper

finely chopped fresh coriander

Cook the rice, drain and rinse under cold running water. Spread the drained rice on a plate, cover and refrigerate until cold. Fry the onion, garlic and chilli in the oil until soft, then add the spices, rice and raisins. Cook for 5 minutes or so, stirring constantly, until heated through. Garnish with chopped coriander.

SALADS

As so much of what is grown in the region is ideal for salads, it's not surprising that Central American cooks have a huge array of salad dishes they prepare regularly. Avocado, beans, corn, hearts of palm, potatoes and quinoa are all particularly popular ingredients and dishes made with them are typically found all over the region.

Salads are normally served as appetisers or as accompaniments to the main course. They are also used to garnish snacks or turned into a main course by using them as a filling or piling them high on tortillas.

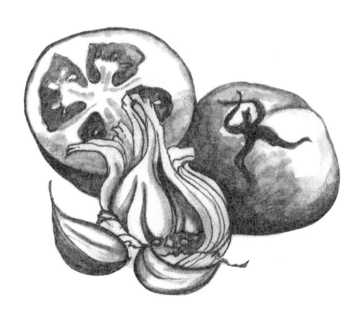

Mayan salad platter

Combinations of fresh fruits and vegetable salad ingredients, arranged on a platter and drizzled with a dressing, are very popular and vary according to what is available locally. Any of the following ingredients can be used to make an authentic salad platter.

avocado slices

roasted sliced peppers

hearts of palm

baby sweetcorn

paw paw slices

diced cooked potatoes

trimmed spring onions

steamed green beans

raw carrot sticks

tomato wedges

onion rings

diced pineapple

sliced banana

cucumber slices

shredded lettuce or spinach leaves

dressing

4 tablespoons olive oil

1 tablespoon white wine vinegar

1 tablespoon lemon or lime juice

1 garlic clove, crushed

black pepper

garnish

chilli rings

chopped fresh coriander

Spread the shredded lettuce or spinach on a platter and top with a selection of salad ingredients arranged in rows. Mix the dressing ingredients together and drizzle over the salad. Garnish with chilli rings and chopped coriander.

Avocado, tomato and corn salad (serves 4)

1 large avocado, peeled, stoned and diced

8oz/225g tomatoes, skinned and chopped

8oz/225g sweetcorn kernels

4 spring onions, trimmed and finely sliced

1 small red chilli, deseeded and finely chopped

1 garlic clove, crushed

1 tablespoon lime juice

dash of Tabasco sauce

black pepper

shredded lettuce leaves

finely chopped fresh parsley

Blanch the sweetcorn kernels, drain and rinse under cold running water. Drain well and mix with the rest of the ingredients apart from the lettuce and parsley. Serve on a bed of shredded lettuce, garnished with chopped parsley.

Vegetable and salsa salad (serves 4)

8oz/225g potatoes, peeled

4oz/100g courgette, diced

4oz/100g baby corn, cut into ½ inch/1cm slices

4oz/100g green beans, topped, tailed and cut into 1 inch/2.5cm lengths

finely chopped fresh parsley

salsa

6oz/175g tomatoes, skinned and finely chopped

2 spring onions, trimmed and finely chopped

1 garlic clove, crushed

½ green chilli, deseeded and finely chopped

1 dessertspoon olive oil

1dessertspoon white wine vinegar

1 teaspoon lemon juice

½ teaspoon dried oregano

black pepper

Cook the potato, drain and rinse under cold water, then dice and put in a mixing bowl. Steam the other vegetables until just tender and rinse under cold running water to refresh. Drain well and add to the potato. Mix all the salsa ingredients until well combined, then add to the vegetables and toss thoroughly. Transfer to a serving bowl, cover and chill for a few hours. Serve garnished with chopped parsley.

Warm cabbage salad (serves 4)

12oz/350g green cabbage

1 small onion, peeled and finely chopped

2 garlic cloves, crushed

2 dessertspoons olive oil

1 dessertspoon white wine vinegar

1 dessertspoon lemon juice

1 teaspoon dried oregano

¼ teaspoon cayenne pepper

black pepper

Mix the olive oil with the vinegar, lemon juice, oregano, cayenne pepper and garlic and season with black pepper. Cut the thick stalks from the cabbage and finely shred the leaves. Bring a large pan of water to the boil, add the shredded cabbage and blanch for 3 minutes. Drain and add the onion and the dressing. Toss well and serve warm.

Potato and bean salad (serves 4)

1lb/450g potatoes, peeled

6oz/175g cooked mixed beans

4oz/100g tomato, peeled and finely chopped

1 small red onion, peeled and finely chopped

1 garlic clove, crushed

1 dessertspoon olive oil

1 tablespoon lemon juice

dash of Tabasco sauce

black pepper

finely chopped fresh parsley

Boil the potatoes, then drain and rinse. Dice them and put them in a large bowl with the beans and onion. Mix the olive oil with the lemon juice and put in another bowl with the tomato, garlic and Tabasco sauce. Season with black pepper and combine well. Add the tomato mixture to the potatoes and beans and toss thoroughly. Spoon into a serving bowl and garnish with chopped parsley.

Roasted pepper and hearts of palm salad (serves 4)

1lb/450g mixed peppers

14oz/400g tin hearts of palm, drained, rinsed and chopped

2oz/50g baby spinach leaves, finely shredded

4 spring onions, trimmed and sliced

1 garlic clove, crushed

1 dessertspoon Dijon mustard

1 dessertspoon olive oil

1 tablespoon lemon juice

black pepper

Roast the peppers under a hot grill until the skins blister. Allow to cool slightly, then carefully remove the skins, stalks, membranes and seeds. Chop the flesh and put it in a bowl with the hearts of palm, spinach and spring onions. Mix the mustard with the olive oil, lemon juice and garlic and season with black pepper. Add to the other ingredients and toss well before transferring the salad to a serving dish. Cover and chill.

Chayote, orange and avocado salad (serves 4)

1 medium chayote, peeled and diced

1 large orange

1 medium avocado, peeled, stoned and diced

1 small bunch of watercress, trimmed

1 rounded tablespoon finely chopped fresh coriander

1 dessertspoon olive oil

1 teaspoon white wine vinegar

pinch of cayenne pepper

black pepper

chopped walnuts

Steam the chayote just long enough to soften it slightly, then rinse under cold running water to refresh. Drain well and put in a mixing bowl with the avocado. Peel the orange and remove the pith, membranes and pips. Chop the segments, drain and keep the juice, and add them to the bowl together with the watercress and coriander. Mix the olive oil, vinegar and cayenne pepper with the orange juice, season with black pepper and pour over the salad. Toss thoroughly, then spoon into a serving dish and scatter chopped walnuts on top.

Bean and tomato salad (serves 4)

8oz/225g cooked mixed beans

8oz/225g green beans, topped, tailed and cut into ½ inch/1cm lengths

7oz/200g tin crushed tomatoes

1 small red onion, peeled and finely chopped

1 garlic clove, crushed

1 rounded tablespoon finely chopped fresh parsley

1 tablespoon lemon juice

¼ teaspoon ground allspice

¼ teaspoon cayenne pepper

black pepper

extra chopped fresh parsley

Steam the green beans until just tender, then refresh under cold water. Drain well and put in a mixing bowl with the cooked beans and the onion. Combine the garlic, parsley, lemon juice, allspice and cayenne pepper with the crushed tomatoes and season with black pepper. Add to the beans and toss thoroughly. Transfer to a serving bowl, cover and chill. Sprinkle with chopped parsley before serving.

Quinoa, chickpea and corn salad (serves 4)

4oz/100g quinoa

8 fl.oz/225ml vegetable stock

4oz/100g tomato, skinned and finely chopped

4oz/100g cooked chickpeas

4oz/100g sweetcorn kernels

2 spring onions, trimmed and finely sliced

1 garlic clove, crushed

1 small green chilli

1 rounded tablespoon finely chopped fresh parsley

1 dessertspoon lime juice

1 dessertspoon olive oil

black pepper

finely grated lime peel

shredded lettuce leaves

Rinse the quinoa and bring it to the boil with the vegetable stock in a small pan. Cover and simmer for about 15 minutes until the liquid has been absorbed. Allow to cool, then refrigerate until cold. Blanch the sweetcorn kernels, rinse under cold running water, drain and put in a bowl with the chickpeas. Cut a few rings from the chilli and keep for garnish. Deseed and finely chop the rest and put in a small bowl with the tomato, spring onions, garlic, parsley, lime juice and oil. Season with black pepper and mix before adding to the chickpeas and corn. Add the cold quinoa and toss well. Arrange some shredded lettuce on a plate and pile the salad on top. Garnish with the chilli rings and some grated lime peel.

Roasted garlic and vegetable salad (serves 4)

8oz/225g potatoes, peeled

6oz/175g baby corn, cut into ½ inch/1cm slices

4oz/100g green beans, topped, tailed and cut into 1 inch/2.5cm
   lengths

4oz/100g shelled peas

4 spring onions, trimmed and finely sliced

1 green chilli

1 rounded tablespoon finely chopped fresh coriander

6 garlic cloves

1 tablespoon olive oil

1 teaspoon olive oil

1 dessertspoon lemon juice

1 dessertspoon white wine vinegar

¼ teaspoon ground cumin

black pepper

shredded spinach leaves

Trim the tops and bottoms from the garlic cloves but leave the papery skins on. Put the cloves in a small pan with the teaspoonful of oil and gently roast them over a medium heat until softened. Carefully remove the skins and crush the cloves. Combine the crushed garlic with the tablespoonful of oil and the lemon juice, vinegar and cumin. Season with black pepper and mix thoroughly.

Boil the potatoes, drain and rinse under cold water, dice and put in a mixing bowl with the spring onions and coriander. Blanch or steam the baby corn cobs, green beans and peas until just tender, then rinse under cold water to refresh. Drain well and add to the bowl. Cut a few rings from the chilli for garnish, deseed and finely chop the remainder and add to the salad together with the garlic dressing. Toss thoroughly, then cover and chill for a few hours. Arrange the shredded spinach leaves on a serving plate, pile the salad on top and garnish with the chilli rings.

Wheat tortilla salad (serves 4)

4 7inch/18cm wheat tortillas (see page 90)
8oz/225g sweet potatoes, peeled and diced
4oz/100g green pepper, chopped
4oz/100g tomato, chopped
4oz/100g baby corn, cut into ½ inch/1cm slices
few crisp lettuce leaves, shredded
1 tablespoon olive oil
1 tablespoon lemon juice
1 dessertspoon chopped drained bottled jalapeño chillies
1 garlic clove, crushed
2 tablespoons finely chopped fresh parsley
black pepper
2 spring onions, trimmed and finely sliced

Steam the potato and rinse under cold running water. Drain well and put in a large bowl with the green pepper and tomato. Blanch the baby corn, rinse under cold water, drain and add together with the lettuce, chillies and half of the parsley. Chop the tortillas into thin strips of about 1 inch/2.5cm long and add to the bowl. Combine the olive oil, lemon juice and garlic and season with black pepper. Pour over the salad and toss well. Spoon into a serving dish and sprinkle with the spring onions and the remaining parsley.

Hearts of palm and corn salad (serves 4)

14oz/400g tin hearts of palm, drained, rinsed and finely chopped

8oz/225g sweetcorn kernels

2oz/50g cucumber, finely chopped

2oz/50g red pepper, finely chopped

2 spring onions, trimmed and finely chopped

2 garlic cloves, crushed

1 tablespoon olive oil

1 dessertspoon lemon juice

1 dessertspoon white wine vinegar

1 teaspoon Dijon mustard

black pepper

shredded lettuce

finely chopped fresh parsley

Blanch the sweetcorn, then rinse under cold water, drain and place in a mixing bowl with the hearts of palm, cucumber, red pepper and spring onions. Mix the olive oil with the lemon juice, vinegar, mustard and garlic. Season with black pepper and add to the salad. Toss thoroughly, then serve on a bed of shredded lettuce, garnished with parsley.

SALSAS AND SAUCES

A Central American cook's repertoire of salsa recipes is literally never-ending and only limited by what fruits and vegetables are readily available or in season. These imaginative, easy-to-make and delicious little dishes are served with every meal as accompaniments and are used as toppings or fillings in other recipes.

Salsas and sauces are generally served in bowls for diners to help themselves to and both are excellent for livening up plainly cooked vegetables or grain dishes and giving them an instant flavour of the region.

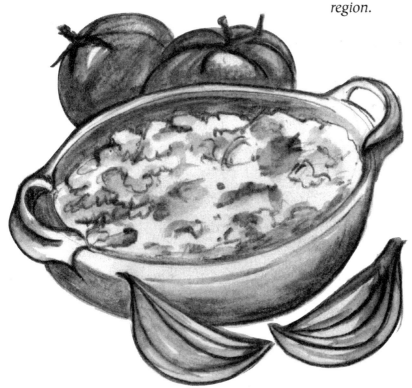

Roasted pepper and garlic salsa (serves 4)

1lb/450g mixed peppers

4 garlic cloves

1 dessertspoon olive oil

1 dessertspoon lemon juice

black pepper

Cut the peppers in half lengthways and remove the stalks, seeds and membranes. Put them on a baking tray, skin side up, under a hot grill until the skins blister. At the same time grill the garlic cloves until soft. Carefully remove the skins from the peppers and finely chop the flesh. Crush the garlic cloves and add to the peppers. Mix the olive oil with the lemon juice and add, then season with black pepper and combine thoroughly. Spoon into a serving bowl, cover and chill before serving.

Pineapple and cucumber salsa (serves 4)

8oz/225g pineapple flesh, finely chopped and drained

2oz/50g cucumber, finely chopped

2 spring onions, trimmed and finely chopped

1 small red chilli, deseeded and finely chopped

1 teaspoon capers, finely chopped

1 tablespoon finely chopped fresh parsley

1 dessertspoon lime juice

black pepper

Mix all the ingredients well, then transfer to a serving bowl. Cover and chill.

Tomato and chilli salsa (serves 4)

12oz/350g tomatoes, skinned and finely chopped

1 red chilli, deseeded and finely chopped

1 garlic clove, crushed

2 spring onions, trimmed and finely chopped

1 dessertspoon lemon juice

1 rounded tablespoon finely chopped fresh coriander

black pepper

Strain the excess juice from the tomatoes, then combine them well with the rest of the ingredients. Cover and chill before serving.

Avocado and tomato salsa (serves 4)

1 medium avocado, peeled, stoned and finely chopped

6oz/175g tomatoes, skinned and finely chopped

1 small red onion, peeled and finely chopped

1 garlic clove, crushed

1 tablespoon lime juice

1 rounded tablespoon finely chopped fresh coriander

black pepper

Mix the ingredients until well combined, then spoon into a serving bowl, cover and chill.

Paw paw and lime sauce (serves 4)

1 paw paw, peeled, deseeded and diced

juice of 1 lime

½oz/15g sultanas

1 small red onion, peeled and finely chopped

½ inch/1cm piece of root ginger, finely chopped

1 garlic clove, crushed

1 dessertspoon sunflower oil

1 tablespoon brown sugar

Fry the onion, ginger and garlic in the oil until soft. Add the remaining ingredients and stir well, then simmer for 10 minutes uncovered, stirring occasionally, until the liquid has been absorbed. Transfer to a bowl, cover and serve chilled.

Pumpkin seed sauce (serves 4)

2oz/50g pumpkin seeds, roasted and ground

1 onion, peeled and chopped

1 green chilli, deseeded and chopped

1 garlic clove

1 tablespoon sunflower oil

2 tablespoons finely chopped fresh coriander

½ teaspoon ground cumin

6 fl.oz/175ml vegetable stock

1 teaspoon cornflour

black pepper

Blend the onion, chilli and garlic smooth, then fry in the oil for 5 minutes and take off the heat. Mix the cornflour with the vegetable stock until smooth and add to the pan with the remaining ingredients. Mix until thoroughly combined, then return the pan to the heat and bring the sauce to the boil while stirring. Continue stirring for a couple of minutes before transferring to a bowl. Serve hot.

Roasted tomato and jalapeño sauce (serves 4)

1lb/450g tomatoes, halved

1 small red onion, peeled and finely chopped

2 garlic cloves, crushed

1 dessertspoon olive oil

1 dessertspoon tomato purée

1 dessertspoon lemon juice

1 tablespoon finely chopped drained bottled jalapeño chillies

½ teaspoon dried oregano

black pepper

Place the tomato halves on a baking tray under a medium hot grill until soft, then carefully remove the skins. Soften the onion and garlic in the oil and put in a blender with the tomatoes, tomato purée, lemon juice and oregano. Season with black pepper and blend smooth. Transfer to a small pan and add the chillies. Gently heat while stirring until the sauce is hot before serving.

Onion escabeche (serves 4)

1lb/450g onions, peeled and thinly sliced

4oz/100g tomato, skinned and thinly sliced

1 green chilli, deseeded and finely chopped

2 dessertspoons olive oil

2 tablespoons white wine vinegar

4 tablespoons water

½ teaspoon ground cumin

black pepper

Fry the onions in the oil, stirring occasionally, for 10 minutes. Add the rest of the ingredients and raise the heat to a simmer. Cook for 5 minutes, stirring frequently until done, then transfer to a serving dish. Serve hot or cold.

BREADS

Corn tortillas have reputedly been made in Central America for at least 7,000 years. Today they are still the most popular form of 'bread' in the region and in many of the countries they are eaten with every meal. These essential accompaniments also find their way into other dishes or are made into a meal in themselves with savoury fillings. Wheat was introduced to the region by the Spaniards in the 16th century and this opened up new possibilities for breadmaking. Tortillas made from wheat are more flexible than those made from corn and can be used in a variety of ways to enclose sweet and savoury fillings.

Cornbread is very popular in all the countries and as well as the recipe featured here, other typical varieties use chopped chillies, peppers or cheese. Johnny cakes are a Caribbean speciality and these are especially popular in Belize, where a large proportion of the population is descended from Carib Indians. French baguette-style bread is commonly found in bakeries all over the region and these are often cut into long lengths 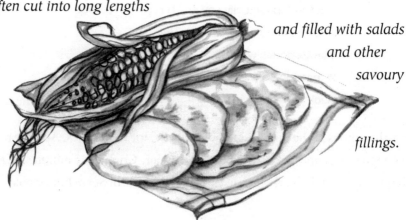 *and filled with salads and other savoury*

fillings.

Corn tortillas (makes 8)

4oz/100g masa harina
pinch of salt
approx. 4 fl.oz/125ml hot water

Mix the masa harina with the salt and gradually add enough water for the mixture to bind and form a soft ball. Care needs to be taken at this stage to ensure that the dough is neither too dry and crumbly nor too wet and sticky. Knead the dough well, then divide into 8 equal portions and roll each one into a ball.

Cut out 16 squares of greaseproof paper measuring 4 inches/10cm . Put a ball of dough in the centre of a piece of greaseproof paper and place another sheet on top, then press down firmly on the dough with the bottom of a saucepan until it is about 3½ inches/9cm in diameter. Repeat with the remaining dough and don't remove the paper until ready to cook.

Heat a heavy-based non-stick frying pan until hot. Carefully peel off one of the pieces of paper and invert the tortilla into the hot pan. Take off the top paper and cook the tortilla for 30-60 seconds until lightly browned underneath, then turn it over and cook the other side. Serve warm, with a savoury topping or as an accompaniment.

Thick 'cheese' tortillas (makes 8)

Add:

1oz/25g grated vegan 'cheese'

to the masa harina and salt as above, then add the water to make the dough and divide this into 8 equal pieces. Press each piece of dough between sheets of greaseproof paper to approximately ¼ inch/5mm thick and cook and serve in the same way as plain corn tortillas.

Wheat tortillas (makes 8)

8oz/225g plain flour

pinch of salt

4 tablespoons corn oil

approx. 3 fl.oz/75ml warm water

Mix the flour with the salt in a large bowl and stir in the oil. Gradually add the water until a soft dough forms. Knead this well on a floured board and divide it into 8 equal pieces. Roll each one into a ball, then roll these out very thinly on a floured board into a circle of about 7 inches/18cm. Keep the tortillas covered with kitchen paper or a clean cloth to prevent them from drying out.

Heat a heavy-based non-stick frying pan until hot and carefully put a tortilla in the pan, making sure it lies flat. Cook for about 40 seconds over a medium heat until lightly speckled brown underneath. Turn the tortilla over and cook the other side. Transfer to a plate and keep covered until all the tortillas are made.

Honduran herbed flat bread (makes 4)

12oz/350g plain flour

1 rounded teaspoon baking powder

pinch of salt

2 tablespoons olive oil

1 rounded teaspoon dried oregano

1 rounded teaspoon dried sage

1 rounded teaspoon dried basil

water

extra olive oil

Mix the flour with the baking powder, salt and herbs. Stir in the olive oil, then add enough water to bind. Knead the dough well and divide it into 4 equal pieces. Roll each of these into a ball and flatten them into 6 inch/15cm circles. Lightly oil a non-stick pan and heat until hot. Cook the breads for a few minutes on each side until golden. Serve warm.

Cornbread

4oz/100g sweetcorn kernels

4oz/100g cornmeal

4oz/100g plain flour

1 rounded teaspoon baking powder

4 tablespoons corn oil

1 small onion, peeled and grated

½ teaspoon paprika

Blanch the sweetcorn kernels, drain over a bowl and blend with 4 fl.oz/125ml of the cooking liquid. Mix the cornmeal with the flour, baking powder and paprika. Stir in the oil, then rub it into the dry ingredients with the fingertips. Add the onion and blended sweetcorn and mix thoroughly. Spoon the dough into a lined and greased 6 inch/15cm square baking tin and level the top, then bake in a preheated oven at 180°C/350°F/Gas mark 4 for about 20 minutes until golden brown. Carefully turn the cornbread out of the tin and serve warm, cut into thick slices.

Johnny cakes (makes 8)

8oz/225g plain flour

1oz/25g vegan margarine, melted

2 teaspoons baking powder

approx. 4 fl.oz/125ml coconut milk

Sift the flour and baking powder into a mixing bowl and stir in the margarine. Combine thoroughly, then gradually add the coconut milk until a stiff dough forms. Knead this well and divide it into 8 equal portions. Roll each one into a ball, flatten these slightly and put them on a greased baking tray. Prick the tops with a fork and bake in a preheated oven at 180°C/350°F/Gas mark 4 for about 20 minutes until golden. Serve warm, sliced open and spread with a savoury topping.

Picos (makes 16)

8oz/225g plain flour

1 teaspoon easy-blend yeast

pinch of salt

1 tablespoon corn oil

approx. 4 fl.oz/125ml warm water

vegan 'Parmesan'

chopped drained bottled jalapeño chillies

Mix the flour with the yeast and salt in a large bowl, stir in the oil and gradually add the water until a soft dough forms. Knead this well, then return it to the bowl, cover and leave in a warm place for 1 hour to rise. Knead the dough again and divide it into 8 equal pieces. Roll each one out on a floured board into a square of about 6 inches/15cm. Cut the squares in half diagonally to make 16 triangles. Sprinkle each triangle with 'Parmesan' and chopped chillies, then dampen the edges of the dough with water. Fold the triangles in half, press the edges together to join and put them on a greased baking sheet in a warm place for 30 minutes. Bake in a preheated oven at 200°C/400°F/Gas mark 6 for 6-8 minutes until browned. Serve warm.

Panamanian fried bread (makes 6)

8oz/225g plain flour

1 rounded teaspoon baking powder

pinch of salt

1oz/25g vegan margarine, melted

approx. 4 fl.oz/125ml water

corn oil

Mix the flour with the baking powder and salt, stir in the melted margarine and gradually add the water until everything binds together. Knead the dough on a floured board and divide it into 6 equal pieces. Roll each piece into a ball and flatten these into circles of about ¼ inch/5mm thick. Heat a small amount of oil in a non-stick pan and fry the rounds for a few minutes on each side until golden brown. Drain on kitchen paper and serve warm.

Chilli and corn buns (makes 8)

4oz/100g plain flour

4oz/100g cornmeal

1 rounded teaspoon baking powder

4oz/100g sweetcorn kernels

4 tablespoons corn oil

1 tablespoon finely chopped drained bottled jalapeño chillies

¼ teaspoon cayenne pepper

Blanch the sweetcorn kernels, drain and keep the cooking liquid. Mix the flour with the cornmeal, baking powder and cayenne pepper in a large bowl, stir in the oil and combine thoroughly. Add the sweetcorn kernels and chillies together with 6 fl.oz/175ml of the cooking liquid. Mix well, then divide the dough between 8 greased holes of a non-stick bun tin. Bake in a preheated oven at 180°C/350°F/Gas mark 4 for 15-18 minutes until golden. Carefully remove the buns from the tin and serve warm.

DESSERTS

Fresh fruit salads are the most commonly served everyday desserts and are usually all that is required to round off the filling main meals served across the region. They are traditionally made from a couple of complementing fruits or from a mixture chosen from the wide variety of exotic fruits that are grown in each of the countries. Other desserts are usually reserved for special occasions or are eaten at other times of the day as snacks.

Dozens of different types of bananas are grown all over Central America, some of which need to be cooked before eating. These varieties are baked, boiled, barbecued or steamed in their skins until tender and then peeled and sprinkled with lime juice, sugar and ground spices such as cinnamon, allspice and cloves.

A wide choice of cold custard-type dishes and sweet rice puddings are found and these are extremely popular in all Latin American countries. Sweetcorn may seem an unusual ingredient in desserts, but not in Central America where it is such a staple and is used for instance to make a delicious, richly-flavoured ice cream.

Mango and paw paw pudding (serves 4)

1 small mango, peeled, stoned and diced

1 paw paw, peeled, deseeded and diced

topping

4oz/100g plain flour

1oz/25g vegan margarine

1oz/25g brown sugar

1 rounded teaspoon baking powder

5 fl.oz/150ml coconut milk

¼ teaspoon ground allspice

Mix the mango with the paw paw and put it in a greased 7 inch/18cm diameter baking dish. Cream the margarine with the sugar, then add the sifted flour and baking powder and allspice alternately with the coconut milk. Mix thoroughly until well combined and spoon the topping evenly over the fruit. Bake in a preheated oven at 180°C/350°F/Gas mark 4 for about 30 minutes until golden. Serve warm, topped with yoghurt or ice cream.

Orange and cinnamon custard cups (serves 4)

10 fl.oz/300ml fresh orange juice

4 inch/10cm stick of cinnamon, crumbled

10 fl.oz/300ml soya milk

1oz/25g brown sugar

1oz/25g cornflour

1 large orange

ground cinnamon

Put the orange juice and cinnamon stick in a small pan and bring to the boil. Cover and simmer for 3 minutes, then remove from the heat. Peel the orange and grate a small piece of the peel for garnish. Remove the membranes and pips from the orange, chop the segments and divide these between 4 glass dishes. Strain the orange juice, discard the cinnamon stick and pour the juice back into the pan. Dissolve the cornflour and sugar in the soya milk and add to the orange juice. Stir well and bring to the boil while stirring, then continue stirring for a minute or so until the custard thickens. Pour the custard over the chopped orange in the dishes and cover and chill for a few hours until set. Sprinkle the grated peel and some ground cinnamon on top before serving.

Guava and ginger sorbet (serves 4)

14oz/400g tin guavas in syrup
1oz/25g fresh root ginger, peeled and finely chopped
5 fl.oz/150ml water

Bring the ginger and water to the boil in a small saucepan. Cover and simmer for 3 minutes, then remove from the heat and allow to cool. Put the guavas and syrup in a blender and add the cooled ginger liquid. Blend smooth and pour into a shallow freezerproof container. Cover and freeze for 1 hour, then whisk the mixture and return it to the freezer for a few hours until just frozen. Keep at room temperature for about 45 minutes before serving if the sorbet freezes too hard.

Spiced raisin rice (serves 4)

4oz/100g long grain rice
2oz/50g raisins
1oz/25g brown sugar
10 fl.oz/300ml water
10 fl.oz/300ml soya milk
2 inch/5cm stick of cinnamon, broken
8 cloves
ground allspice

Put the rice, water, cinnamon and cloves in a pan and bring to the boil. Cover and simmer gently until the liquid has been absorbed. Remove from the heat and discard the cinnamon and cloves, then add the raisins, sugar and soya milk and stir well. Return to the stove and bring back to the boil. Cover and simmer gently until the soya milk has been absorbed. Divide the rice between 4 serving glasses and serve warm, sprinkled with ground allspice.

Baked sweet potato pudding (serves 4)

1lb/450g sweet potatoes, peeled and grated

2oz/50g raisins

1oz/25g brown sugar

8 fl.oz/225ml coconut milk

1 teaspoon vanilla essence

ground cinnamon

Bring all the ingredients apart from the cinnamon to the boil in a saucepan, then transfer to a baking dish. Cover and bake in a preheated oven at 180°C/350°F/Gas mark 4 for 30 minutes. Serve hot, lightly sprinkled with ground cinnamon.

Banana with chilled mocha custard (serves 4)

2 ripe bananas, peeled and chopped

lemon juice

6 fl.oz/175ml black coffee

8 fl.oz/225ml soya milk

1oz/25g dark vegan chocolate bar, broken

1 rounded tablespoon cornflour

1 rounded tablespoon brown sugar

½ teaspoon vanilla essence

¼ teaspoon ground allspice

grated dark vegan chocolate bar

Divide the bananas between 4 glass dishes and sprinkle them with lemon juice.

Put the coffee, broken chocolate bar, sugar, vanilla and ground allspice in a double boiler and heat gently until the chocolate melts. Mix the cornflour with the soya milk until smooth and add to the pan. Combine thoroughly, then bring to the boil, stirring constantly, until the custard thickens. Remove from the heat and continue stirring for a minute or so until the mixture becomes very smooth. Pour the custard over the banana, cover and refrigerate until set. Sprinkle grated chocolate on top when serving.

Iced sweetcorn cream (serves 4)

12oz/350g sweetcorn kernels

6 fl.oz/175ml water

9 fl.oz/250ml vegan 'cream'

1 teaspoon vanilla essence

1 tablespoon brown sugar

Put the sweetcorn and water in a pan and bring to the boil. Cover and simmer for 3 minutes, then transfer to a blender and blend to a purée. Pass this through a fine sieve, pressing out as much as possible with the back of a spoon to leave only the skins in the sieve. Add the 'cream', vanilla and sugar to the purée and combine well. Pour the mixture into a shallow freezerproof container, cover and freeze for 1 hour, then whisk it and return it to the freezer for a few hours until just set. If the ice freezes too hard, transfer it to room temperature for about 45 minutes before serving.

Mango and coconut cups (serves 4)

1 large ripe mango, peeled and diced

2 fl.oz/50ml water

1 tablespoon brown sugar

8 fl.oz/225ml thin coconut milk

1 tablespoon cornflour

toasted flaked coconut

Put 6oz/175g of mango in a small pan with the water and sugar. Bring to the boil, cover and simmer until the fruit is pulpy. Divide the remaining mango between 4 serving dishes. Mix the cornflour with 2 fl.oz/50ml of the coconut milk until smooth. Blend the cooked mango with the rest of the coconut milk. Pour into a small saucepan and add the cornflour mixture. Mix thoroughly, then bring to the boil while stirring and continue stirring for a minute or so until the mixture thickens. Pour the custard over the fruit in the dishes, cover and chill. Serve sprinkled with flaked coconut.

Banana and peanut ice cream (serves 4)

8oz/225g ripe bananas, peeled and chopped

9 fl.oz/250ml vegan 'cream'

2 rounded tablespoons peanut butter

1 teaspoon vanilla essence

lemon juice

Sprinkle the banana with lemon juice and blend it smooth with the remaining ingredients. Pour into a shallow freezerproof container, cover and freeze for 1 hour. Whisk the mixture thoroughly, then return to the freezer for a few hours until frozen. If the ice cream becomes too hard, keep it at room temperature for about 45 minutes before serving.

Grapefruit and guava salad (serves 4)

1 red-fleshed grapefruit

14oz/400g tin guavas in syrup

grated creamed coconut

Peel the grapefruit and remove the pith, membranes and pips. Chop the segments and put them in a mixing bowl. Cut the guava halves into quarters and add to the grapefruit together with the syrup. Mix well, then divide between 4 serving glasses. Cover and chill, and sprinkle with grated creamed coconut to serve.

BAKING

Central Americans are
generally very keen on cakes
and biscuits and these
are enjoyed with coffee
or hot chocolate drinks
at any time of the day.
With sugarcane being
a major agricultural
crop in all seven countries,
sugar is cheap and plentiful
and added liberally in sweet
recipes. In fact, most recipes
would be far too sweet for
all but those with the sweetest
tooth elsewhere, so in the interest of
both taste and health the recipes included here
contain only a fraction of the sugar that would be
added in Central American countries. Not
surprisingly, sweetcorn finds its way into a cake
recipe, and cakes containing fresh fruits are also very
popular. Sweet empanadas are widely found and these
can easily be made with the pastry from the savoury empanadas recipe
on page 63, using mashed or chopped banana with raisins and
chopped nuts as a filling. Other typical sweet dishes include fruit pies
or flans made with mango or paw paw and cooked pastry flan cases
filled with set fruit custard.

Carrot bread

9oz/250g plain flour

8oz/225g carrots, scraped and grated

2oz/50g raisins

2oz/50g brown sugar

4 fl.oz/125ml sunflower oil

5 fl.oz/150ml fresh orange juice

1 rounded tablespoon golden syrup

1 rounded teaspoon baking powder

1 teaspoon ground cinnamon

1 teaspoon vanilla essence

sesame seeds

Mix the sugar with the oil, golden syrup and vanilla in a large bowl until well combined. Stir in the carrots and raisins, then add the sifted flour and baking powder and the cinnamon alternately with the orange juice. Mix thoroughly and spoon into a base-lined and greased 8 inch/20cm loaf tin. Sprinkle the top with sesame seeds, cover and bake in a preheated oven at 180°C/350°F/Gas mark 4 for 25 minutes. Uncover and bake for a further 20-25 minutes until the bread is golden brown and a skewer comes out clean when inserted in the centre. Run a sharp knife around the edges to loosen, then carefully turn out onto a wire rack and allow to cool before cutting into slices.

Spiced cornmeal cookies (makes approx. 24)

4oz/100g cornmeal

2oz/50g plain flour

2oz/50g vegan margarine

2oz/50g brown sugar

1 teaspoon baking powder

1 teaspoon ground allspice

½ teaspoon vanilla essence

4 tablespoons soya milk

Cream the margarine with the sugar and vanilla essence, stir in the cornmeal, sifted flour and baking powder and the allspice and mix until crumbly. Add the soya milk and stir well until everything binds together. Take heaped teaspoonfuls of the mixture and roll into balls. Flatten these into small biscuit shapes and indent the tops with a fork. Bake in a preheated oven at 180°C/350°F/Gas mark 4 for 15-18 minutes until golden. Slide onto a wire rack to cool.

Honduran spiced bun

8oz/225g plain flour

2oz/50g brown sugar

1oz/25g vegan margarine, melted

1 rounded teaspoon easy-blend yeast

1 teaspoon ground cinnamon

½ teaspoon ground allspice

approx. 5 fl.oz/150ml warm water

extra ground cinnamon and allspice

Mix the flour with the sugar, yeast, teaspoonful ground cinnamon and ½ teaspoonful ground allspice in a mixing bowl. Stir in the margarine, then gradually add the water until a soft dough forms. Knead the dough well, return it to the bowl, cover and leave in a warm place for 1 hour to rise. Knead the dough again, then roll it into a 'sausage' shape, measuring about 24 inches/61cm. Brush the top of the roll with water and sprinkle with ground cinnamon and allspice. Roll the 'sausage' up in a spiral, with the sprinkled spices on the inside. Place the ring on a greased baking sheet and flatten it slightly. Leave in a warm place for 30 minutes, then bake in a preheated oven at 200°C/400°F/Gas mark 6 for 15-20 minutes until browned and hollow sounding when tapped underneath. Allow to cool slightly before cutting into slices.

Peanut and rice cookies (makes 10)

2oz/50g rice flour

2oz/50g plain flour

1oz/25g brown sugar

1 rounded tablespoon peanut butter

1 tablespoon groundnut oil

1 teaspoon baking powder

¼ teaspoon ground cinnamon

3 tablespoons soya milk

Put the sugar, peanut butter and oil in a large bowl and stir until well combined. Add the rice flour and sifted flour, baking powder and cinnamon and mix until crumbly. Add the soya milk and combine thoroughly until everything binds together. Take rounded dessertspoonfuls of the mixture and roll into balls in the palm of the hand, then flatten each ball into a biscuit shape and put them on a greased baking sheet. Prick the tops with a fork and bake in a preheated oven at 180°C/350°F/Gas mark 4 for 12-15 minutes until golden brown. Transfer to a wire rack to cool.

Paw paw and coconut buns (makes 12)

1 paw paw, peeled, deseeded and mashed

6oz/175g plain flour

2oz/50g rice flour

2oz/50g vegan margarine

2oz/50g brown sugar

1 rounded teaspoon baking powder

¼ teaspoon ground allspice

4 fl.oz/125ml coconut milk

Cream the margarine with the sugar and stir in the rice flour. Add first the paw paw and then the sifted flour, baking powder and allspice alternately with the coconut milk. Mix thoroughly, then divide the dough between 12 holes of a non-stick greased bun tin. Bake in a pre-heated oven at 180°C/350°F/Gas mark 4 for 30 minutes. Allow to cool in the tin for 15 minutes, then carefully remove the buns from the tin and serve warm or cold.

Chocolate and brazil nut slices (makes 10)

4oz/100g plain flour

2oz/50g cornflour

2oz/50g brazil nuts, grated

2oz/50g brown sugar

2oz/50g vegan margarine

½oz/15g cocoa powder

1 rounded teaspoon baking powder

1 teaspoon vanilla essence

7 fl.oz/200ml soya milk

1oz/25g dark vegan chocolate bar

chopped brazil nuts

Cream the margarine with the sugar and vanilla essence in a mixing bowl and stir in the cornflour and grated brazil nuts. Add the sifted flour, baking powder and cocoa and mix until crumbly, then add the soya milk and combine thoroughly. Spoon the mixture into a base-lined and greased 7 inch/18cm square baking tin and level the top. Bake in a preheated oven at 180°C/350°F/Gas mark 4 for 25 minutes. Run a sharp knife around the edges to loosen and carefully transfer to a wire rack to cool.

Melt the chocolate bar in a bowl over a pan of boiling water, then spread evenly over the top of the cake. Sprinkle with chopped brazil nuts and chill for a couple of hours until the chocolate sets. Cut the cake in half and each half into 5 equal slices.

Pineapple and coconut cake

8oz/225g tin pineapple rings in natural juice

8oz/225g plain flour

2oz/50g vegan margarine

2oz/50g brown sugar

1oz/25g creamed coconut, grated

1 rounded tablespoon golden syrup

1 tablespoon soya milk

2 rounded teaspoons baking powder

½ teaspoon ground allspice

desiccated coconut

Put the margarine, sugar, creamed coconut and golden syrup in a large pan and heat gently until melted and well combined. Remove from the heat and stir in half of the sifted flour, baking powder and allspice. Finely chop the pineapple rings and put in the pan together with the juice. Add the remaining sifted flour, baking powder and allspice and the soya milk and mix thoroughly. Spoon the mixture into a base-lined and greased 7 inch/18cm round baking tin and level the top. Sprinkle with desiccated coconut, cover and bake in a preheated oven at 180°C/350°F/Gas mark 4 for 30 minutes. Uncover and bake for 15-18 minutes more until browned. Run a sharp knife around the edge to loosen, then carefully turn out onto a wire rack and allow to cool before cutting.

Rum-soaked raisin and mocha cakes (makes 9)

8oz/225g plain flour

2oz/50g raisins, chopped

2oz/50g brown sugar

½oz/15g cocoa powder

4 fl.oz/125ml sunflower oil

5 fl.oz/150ml black coffee

2 tablespoons dark rum

1 rounded tablespoon golden syrup

2 teaspoons baking powder

1 teaspoon vanilla essence

½ teaspoon ground allspice

Soak the raisins in the rum for 2 hours. Gently heat the oil, sugar, golden syrup, cocoa powder and vanilla essence in a large pan until melted and well combined. Remove from the heat and stir in the raisins and any remaining rum. Add the sifted flour, baking powder and allspice alternately with the coffee and mix well. Divide the mixture equally between 9 greased holes of a non-stick bun tin. Bake in a preheated oven at 180°C/350°F/Gas mark 4 for 20-25 minutes until springy to the touch. Allow to cool in the tin for 10 minutes, then put onto a wire rack.

Sweetcorn and sesame cake

4oz/100g sweetcorn kernels

4oz/100g plain flour

2oz/50g sesame seeds, roasted and ground

2oz/50g cornmeal

2oz/50g vegan margarine

2oz/50g brown sugar

5 fl.oz/150ml soya milk

1 rounded teaspoon baking powder

½ teaspoon vanilla essence

sesame seeds

Cream the margarine with the sugar and vanilla essence, then stir in the ground sesame seeds. Blend the sweetcorn kernels with the soya milk and add to the bowl alternately with the sifted flour and baking powder. Now add the cornmeal and combine thoroughly, then spoon the mixture into a base-lined and greased 7 inch/18cm diameter baking tin. Level the top and sprinkle with sesame seeds. Bake in a preheated oven at 180°C/350°F/Gas mark 4 for 25-30 minutes until golden. Run a sharp knife around the edge to loosen, then carefully transfer to a wire rack and allow to cool before cutting.

Banana and peanut cake

6oz/175g ripe bananas, peeled and chopped

6oz/175g plain flour

2 fl.oz/50ml sunflower oil

2oz/50g brown sugar

1 rounded tablespoon peanut butter

1 rounded teaspoon baking powder

½ teaspoon ground cinnamon

lemon juice

5 fl.oz/150ml soya milk

chopped peanuts

Put the oil, sugar and peanut butter in a saucepan, heat gently until well combined, then remove from the heat. Sprinkle the banana with lemon juice, mash and add to the pan. Add the sifted flour, baking powder and cinnamon alternately with the soya milk and mix thoroughly. Spoon the mixture into a base-lined and greased 7 inch/18cm loaf tin and level the top. Sprinkle with chopped peanuts and press these in lightly with the back of a spoon. Cover and bake in a preheated oven at 180°C/350°F/Gas mark 4 for 30 minutes. Uncover and bake for another 10-15 minutes, until the cake is golden brown and a skewer comes out clean when inserted in the middle. Run a sharp knife around the edges to loosen, then carefully turn out onto a wire rack to cool before cutting into slices.

DRINKS

As well as being one of Central America's major exports, coffee is undoubtedly the region's favourite hot drink and copious amounts are enjoyed throughout the day by young and old alike. Such is its popularity that many families ensure they won't go without by growing their own supply of coffee beans in their garden vegetable plots. Coffee is typically served in small cups, either black or white, invariably sweetened and sometimes flavoured with spices such as cinnamon or allspice. Hot chocolate is another popular drink, which originated in Mexico and quickly spread to other countries in Central America. Champurrado, a combination of both coffee and chocolate, is sometimes found thickened with cornmeal rather than cornflour, which gives it a slightly 'gritty' texture.

As in all tropical countries, refreshing cold drinks made from all kinds of fruits offer a welcome respite from the heat and these are regularly made at home or bought ready-made or to order from roadside vendors.

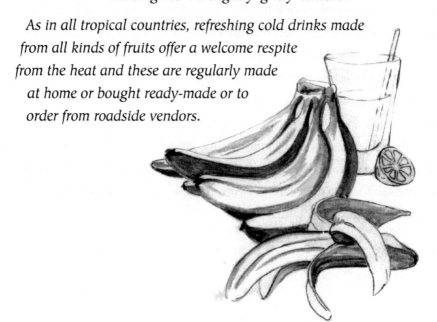

Banana and mango batidos (serves 4)

> 4oz/100g ripe banana, peeled and chopped
>
> 4oz/100g ripe mango flesh, chopped
>
> 1 dessertspoon brown sugar
>
> dash of lime juice
>
> 14 fl.oz/425ml chilled soya milk
>
> 8 fl.oz/225ml chilled water
>
> crushed ice

Blend the banana and mango with the sugar, lime juice and soya milk until smooth. Add the water and mix well, then pour into glasses and add crushed ice.

Tomato and avocado cocktail (serves 4)

> 8oz/225g ripe tomatoes, skinned and chopped
>
> 1 small avocado, peeled, stoned and chopped
>
> 20 fl.oz/600ml water
>
> 1 rounded teaspoon tomato purée
>
> 1 tablespoon lemon juice
>
> dash of Tabasco sauce
>
> crushed ice

Put the tomatoes, tomato purée and half of the water in a pan and bring to the boil. Cover and simmer for 5 minutes, then pass the mixture through a fine sieve, pressing out as much pulp and juice as possible with the back of a spoon so that only the seeds remain in the sieve. Refrigerate the tomato juice until cold, then blend it with the avocado, remaining water, lemon juice and Tabasco sauce until smooth. Pour into glasses and add crushed ice.

Strawberry wine punch (serves 4)

2oz/50g fresh strawberries, chopped
14 fl.oz/425ml chilled red wine
10 fl.oz/300ml soda water
5 fl.oz/150ml chilled fresh orange juice
sliced strawberries
crushed ice

Blend the chopped strawberries smooth with the orange juice, then pass through a sieve into a jug. Add the red wine and soda water and mix well. Put sliced strawberries and crushed ice in each glass when serving.

Paw paw, ginger and apple juice (serves 4)

1 ripe paw paw, peeled, deseeded and chopped
2 inch/5cm piece of root ginger, finely chopped
14 fl.oz/425ml water
10 fl.oz/300ml chilled fresh apple juice
½oz/15g brown sugar
crushed ice

Bring the ginger, sugar and water to the boil. Simmer for 3 minutes, then blend with the paw paw until smooth. Chill the mixture until cold, add the apple juice and whisk thoroughly. Add crushed ice to serve.

Guava and citrus licuados (serves 4)

14oz/400g tin guavas in syrup
1 grapefruit
12 fl.oz/350ml chilled fresh orange juice
crushed ice

Peel the grapefruit and remove the pith, membranes and pips. Chop the segments and put them in a blender with the tinned guavas and syrup. Blend smooth, then pass the mixture through a sieve into a large jug. Add the orange juice and stir well. Pour into glasses and add crushed ice

Pineapple and rice cocktail (serves 4)

22 fl.oz/650ml chilled fresh pineapple juice

1oz/25g long grain rice

8 fl.oz/225ml water

pineapple cubes

Put the rice and water in a small saucepan and bring to the boil. Cover and simmer for 20 minutes, then remove from the heat and refrigerate until cold. Blend the cold rice and cooking liquid smooth with the pineapple juice and pour into glasses. Top each drink with a few pineapple cubes.

Apricot, orange and ginger refrescos (serves 4)

4oz/100g dried apricots, finely chopped

1 inch/2.5cm piece of root ginger, finely chopped

20 fl.oz/600ml water

8 fl.oz/225ml chilled fresh orange juice

crushed ice

Bring the apricots, ginger and water to the boil, cover and simmer for 10 minutes, then blend smooth. Put in the fridge to get cold, then add the orange juice and mix thoroughly. Add some crushed ice to each glass when serving.

Guatemalan champurrado (serves 4)

1oz/25g dark vegan chocolate, chopped

10 fl.oz/300ml black coffee

1 teaspoon vanilla essence

2 rounded dessertspoons brown sugar

½ teaspoon ground cinnamon

16 fl.oz/475ml soya milk

1 rounded dessertspoon cornflour

extra ground cinnamon

grated dark vegan chocolate

Put the chopped chocolate, coffee, vanilla essence, sugar and ½ teaspoonful of cinnamon in a pan and heat gently until the chocolate melts. Mix the cornflour with the soya milk until smooth, then add to the pan and combine well. Bring to the boil while stirring and continue stirring for 1 minute. Remove from the heat and whisk thoroughly before pouring into cups or glasses. Sprinkle with ground cinnamon and grated chocolate and serve immediately.